LEARN THE FACTS—
AND FALLACIES—ABOUT
HAIR LOSS

FACT: *Geographical and cultural influences may affect hormones.* Compared to Asian men, Americans have more of the enzyme that converts testosterone to DHT, and thus have more body hair and more baldness.

MYTH: *The gene for male pattern baldness comes only from the mother.* The truth is that the gene may be passed to a child from either parent, not just the mother, as previously believed.

FACT: *Hair loss is seasonal.* Hair grows most in the spring, when testosterone levels are lowest; and hair loss accelerates in the fall, when testosterone levels peak. Twice as much hair is lost in the fall as in the spring.

FACT: *Diet can affect hair loss.* There is a connection between balding and eating animal fat—particularly red meat—because high fat diets lead to more DHT production and more damage to hair follicles.

Learn what works, what doesn't, what's safe, and what isn't—in the book that shatters the myths and lays bare the facts:

THE BALD TRUTH

THE

BALD TRUTH

THE FIRST COMPLETE GUIDE TO PREVENTING AND TREATING HAIR LOSS

Spencer David Kobren

UPDATED WITH NEW INFORMATION

POCKET BOOKS
New York   London   Toronto   Sydney   Singapore

The author of this book is not a physician, and the ideas, procedures, and suggestions in this book are not intended as a substitute for the medical advice of a trained health professional. All matters regarding your health require medical supervision. Consult your physician before adopting the suggestions in this book, as well as about any condition that may require diagnosis or medical attention. [In addition, the statements made by the author regarding certain products and services represent the views of the author alone, and do not constitute a recommendation or endorsement of any product or service by the publisher.] The author and publisher disclaim any liability arising directly or indirectly from the use of the book [or of any products mentioned herein].

POCKET BOOKS, a division of Simon & Schuster Inc.
1230 Avenue of the Americas, New York, NY 10020

Copyright © 1998 by Spencer David Kobren

Originally published in mass market paperback in 1998 by Pocket Books

Library of Congress Cataloging-in-Publication Data

Kobren, Spencer David.
    The bald truth : the first complete guide to preventing and treating hair loss / Spencer David Kobren.
        p.   cm.
    ISBN: 0-671-04763-9
    Previously published: New York : Pocket Books, 1998.
    Includes bibliographical references.
    1. Baldness—Popular works.   I. Title.

RL155.K63   2000
616.5'46—dc21   00-032682

First Pocket Books trade paperback printing March 2000

10 9 8 7 6 5 4 3 2

POCKET and colophon are registered trademarks of Simon & Schuster Inc.

Printed in the U.S.A.

"In almost all the group interviews where men gathered with me to discuss the ups and downs of middle life, the conversation began with their hair.

"It would seem from the intensity of their concern that losing their hair is for men the first public sign of weakening, almost like walking around with an exposed ego wound that everyone can see, as if hair were what Samson believed it to be: the symbol of a man's power or sexual prowess."

— Gail Sheehy, *New Passages*

To the memory of my mother, Doris Kobren, who provided me with her unconditional love and undying faith

To my father, Jack Kobren, who provided me with his wisdom and everything else

To my big brother, Alan Kobren, who taught me the true meaning of fortitude and tenacity

And to the tens of millions of men and women suffering with the emotional devastation of hair loss

ACKNOWLEDGMENTS

A ten-year journey led to the first edition of *The Bald Truth*. And now, nearly two years later, the journey has only intensified and become more rewarding as I am able to provide information to so many men and women with my weekly syndicated radio program, "The Bald Truth," and with this second edition of the book.

My lifelong friend, Daniel Paige, has given me strength, inspiration and insight, as have Patricia Lynn Johnson, Rafael Raffaelli, III, and Orhan Secilmis. I thank them all so much.

Special thanks to Dr. Angela Christiano, for her continued support of my work, and for her generous friendship; to Dr. Nobel Endicott, who provided me with sound advice and who shared in my vision; and Diane B. Eisman, M.D. and Eugene Eisman, M.D. for their foreword.

Thank you Barbara Brody, Craig Brody, Susan Paige, Joe Gisondi, Janet Firth, Adrian Ball, Ben McGlinn, Lilian Balzana, Brad Brooks, Neil a.k.a. Ross, Betty Allen, Sandy Lebowitz, Hiram Wilson, Louis Salizonni, Jesse O'Kane, Brian Klosenski, Jeff Barton, Richard McRae, Don Randall, Brian Taylor, Nancy Thompson, Marcus Braxton, Julie Rubin, Erica and Alan Rauzin, Pam Johnson, Gary Wilson, Byron Frohman, and all those who have shared their experiences with me by mail, phone, E-mail, and during the call-in segments of my radio program.

Continued thanks to Farrell Manne, who designed *The Bald Truth* website, and who has given of his time and expertise in so many other vital areas.

My deepest gratitude to Robert M. Bernstein, M.D., William R. Rassman, M.D., O'Tar Norwood, M.D., Ron Shapiro, M.D., Bernard Nusbaum, M.D., Bobby L. Limmer, M.D., Roy Jones, M.D., Robert Lehr, M.D., Paul T. Ross, M.D., Robert McClellan, M.D., Bradley Wolf, M.D., Michael Beehner, M.D., and Dr. Barry Sears for their valuable contributions and continued support of my work as a patient and consumer advocate.

Thanks to my radio producer and friend, Peter Bartholomew, and also to the terrific radio crew, including Dennis Cattlett, Tony Dee and Brian Dee.

Thanks to my agent, Frank Curtis, my editor, Mitchell Ivers, managing editor Julie Blattberg and the remarkable staff at Pocket.

My heartfelt thanks to my "hair loss brethren" who have had the courage to share their experiences with the world in this book.

And finally, a very special thank you to journalist and author Nina L. Diamond, who guided me—and this book—through the publishing world and who helped me bring the words out of my head and onto the page.

CONTENTS

CONTENTS

AUTHOR'S NOTE

This book is the result of extensive research, interviews, and reporting. It reports the facts. Those medical treatments it speaks of favorably have been shown to be effective through scientific study and clinical application and have been reported as such by the international scientific community.

The author's opinions do not contradict any of the scientific and medical facts reported here.

FOREWORD

by Diane Batshaw Eisman, M.D.,
and Eugene H. Eisman, M.D.

Baldness is the quiet social stigma. Nobody whispers to their friend at a cocktail party, "Look! Over there . . . near the shredded shrimp in hot sauce . . . a bald man! Ugh!" Yet many people with thinning hair spend hours in front of a mirror devising hairstyles, cluttering up their bathrooms with "cures," or trying to convince themselves they don't care.

It's been a long time since we relied on hair for warmth, and the time is not measured in centuries, but millennia. In the modern world, a hat and coat are more practical for warmth than body hair. But only a few of us have the ego strength to say "So what if I go bald? If my head gets cold, I'll wear a hat!"

In the United States more than 70 million people suffer from male pattern baldness, and the number is rising. Worldwide, the number is staggering. Americans alone spend more than $7 billion a year on hair-loss treatments and restoration. By their late thirties, nearly two-thirds of men become aware of losing their hair.

We are physicians actively involved with the care of our patients. And we are also medical journalists. So we are well aware of how people can be misled, ripped off, and even made to suffer physical damage from marketers of hair-loss products and restoration procedures.

Spencer David Kobren has suffered with hair loss. He's been through it all himself. He is a dedicated hair-loss consumer and patient advocate who provides valuable information that enlightens, guides, and protects men and women who want to safely and effectively prevent and treat hair loss. Among those he's helped, he's been called the "Ralph Nader of hair."

Indeed, Spencer is responsible for an enormous breakthrough in informing the public: this book you are holding.

In *The Bald Truth,* he teaches you how to be your own consumer and patient advocate. His advocacy is also more than welcome in the minds of those leading surgeons you'll read about in Chapter Four who are calling for change within their own hair-transplantation field.

The Bald Truth brings you the best of both mainstream and natural approaches to hair-loss prevention and treatment, and it helps you to distinguish the effective from the hype. By adding this book to your library, you are taking a giant step toward becoming an educated patient and consumer.

Our practice is in the field of internal medicine, cardiology, and family medicine. We encourage our patients to be informed partners in their health care. We have patients—both men and women—who have concerns about hair loss. A person's first medical conversation about this is often with their family doctor, who can guide them through the process of determining effective preventions and treatments and finding medical specialists when needed.

There is so much information available to patients. You can go to your own doctor well informed, comfortable, and knowing what questions to ask. You and your doctor can incorporate the best of mainstream medicine and the best of alternative medicine.

The psychological impact of going bald cannot be underestimated. It is a sign of loss of youth for both men and women. Charlatans have jumped at the opportunity to reap the rewards, and the layperson is their victim.

With *The Bald Truth,* Spencer David Kobren has created an essential guide to keep the unwary out of the hands of the snake-oil people.

FOREWORD

Diane Batshaw Eisman, M.D.
Family Medicine
Miami, Florida
Adjunct Clinical Faculty
University of Miami School of Medicine

Eugene H. Eisman, M.D.
Internal Medicine and Cardiology
Miami, Florida
Adjunct Clinical Faculty
University of Miami School of Medicine

February 1998

——— THE ———
BALD TRUTH

1

THE ROAD TO PROPECIA
Discovering the Cause and Treatment of Baldness

Innovation is not a random process. When
it works, it works because someone has
identified a real need and found a way to
bring new ideas or new technologies to
bear on that need.

—LEWIS W. LEHR

Ask any balding man when he first noticed his hair
thinning, and odds are he'll remember. Like any
other milestone in his life, he isn't likely to forget
the event or its accompanying details, like where
he was, what he was doing, and, most important,
how he felt.

I was in bed, stretching and getting comfortable on the pillow, just like any other night. What

1

made this one different, though, was that when I ran my fingers through my hair, out came, not one or two, but at least ten strands of hair. I couldn't miss it because my hair was worn well below my collar, so these were long strands; a man with shorter hair might not as easily notice the earliest stages of hair loss. I was "lucky."

My heart sank because when this happened, in February 1987, I was only twenty-two. Not that I wouldn't have still been upset had the balding process begun in my thirties or forties, but at twenty-two, with my adult life just beginning, the last thing I wanted to worry about was losing my hair.

The next morning, while in the shower, I noticed that the drain was completely clogged—with my hair. I had a thick head of finely textured hair, and now I was faced with the possibility of losing it to male pattern baldness.

First I tried the then widely advertised Helsinki Formula, then KeraKare, a lotion that's applied to the scalp every night. Neither worked. In fact, some of the over-the-counter topical treatments that used to be marketed as baldness cures disappeared in the wake of the FDA ruling that a product couldn't advertise itself as a hair-loss treatment unless it had specific FDA approval as a hair drug. Yet many of these useless concoctions are still advertised and flood the market because of ineffective enforcement of the law. For seven years I unsuccessfully experimented with every treatment on the market. I found that I really had two "careers." While running my video-production company, Spence-Comm, Inc., I was on an equally time-consuming quest to save my hair. Not only did I spend hours rubbing my head with lotions, I also had "top" New York dermatologists inject hormones into my scalp at $175 per very painful injection. I researched the biological effects of pulsed electrostatic-field treatment for hair, which turned out to be one of the biggest disappointments in the industry. Then, like so many other hopeful men, I ended up using minoxidil, which was then available by prescription only but would eventually be marketed over-the-counter as Rogaine.

A so-called "prominent hair specialist" in New York City was providing me with his own concoction of minoxidil and Retin-A, and he told me to spray this on my scalp four times a day in order to grow hair. According to him, I was the perfect candidate for his potion: I was in my mid-twenties then and my hair loss was not that extensive. My crown was beginning to thin, and my hairline had receded by about half an inch. But I was losing a tremendous amount of hair every day; the balding process was progressing very quickly.

The First Approved Hair Loss Drug

Minoxidil (*loniten*) was the first drug approved by the FDA for treatment of baldness. For many years, minoxidil, in pill form, was widely used to treat high blood pressure. It had one strange side effect, though: It grew hair in an unexpected manner. People grew hair on the backs of their hands, or on their cheeks, and some even grew hair on their foreheads.

Some enterprising researchers had the notion that applying minoxidil topically, directly on the head, might grow hair on balding areas. It did, in varying degrees depending upon the extent of hair loss, and at the time it was revolutionary.

Like all legitimate hair loss treatments, minoxidil works in varying degrees, depending on many hair loss factors. Now marketed over-the-counter under the brand name Rogaine, at the standard 2% solution or the extra strength 5% solution, the drug's side effects include dry, itching or flaking scalp (which is the most common, but easily reduced or eliminated by using common over-the-counter dandruff shampoos like Neutragena

T-Gel, Head and Shoulders or Nizoral), and low blood pressure (which is rare and reversible once you stop using the drug). Minoxidil is not advised, however, for anyone who has heart disease because of the potential for cardiac side effects in those people at risk.

The most recent studies show that Rogaine Extra Strength for men (5% solution) regrew 45% more hair than regular strength Rogaine (2% solution). In the same group of studies, hair regrowth that was shown in month four while using regular strength was visible by month two while using extra strength. This indicates that Rogaine Extra Strength actually speeds up the hair growth process, making treatment that much more effective.

Rogaine is thought to work by stimulating and enlarging miniaturized hair follicles and reversing the miniaturization process. According to Pharmacia & Upjohn, which manufactures and markets Rogaine, regrowth is more likely to occur if you have a large number of only partially miniaturized hair follicles. These kinds of follicles still produce hair, but this hair will be thinner than unaffected strands, and must be at least 3/8 of an inch or more in length for it to favorably respond to Rogaine.

Unfortunately, according to Pharmacia & Upjohn, any area of your scalp with no hair or where only vellus (peach fuzz) hair remains is less likely to respond to treatment. Rogaine is the most effec-

5

tive for the earliest stages of hair loss. The manufacturer also cautions that Rogaine should not be used by those under 18 years of age; those using a topical prescription product on the scalp; those experiencing sunburned, inflamed, infected, irritated or painful scalp; or those whose hair loss was sudden, indicating that it is not male pattern baldness, but some other form of hair loss.

Rogaine's effectiveness can be enhanced by simultaneously using other treatments, including Propecia, herbal, and nutritional approaches. Some men with sensitive scalps do not make good candidates for treatment with Rogaine, and once those men stop using the drug, their scalp irritation will go away.

The DHT Connection and Finasteride

By late 1994, I had amassed quite an amount of information on baldness, so when I read in the *New York Times* that a number of drug companies had committed to putting the next baldness breakthrough on pharmacy shelves, I was intrigued that among the drugs that were being studied was finasteride, the prescription prostate drug that Merck & Co., the pharmaceutical company, manufactured and marketed in a 5 mg. dose under the brand name Proscar. Finasteride prevents testosterone from converting into DHT (dihydrotestosterone), the androgen that can cause not only prostate problems but the demise of hair follicles. I knew from my reading about testosterone that Merck was on to something. Only a product that changes the body's chemistry, introduced internally (with a pill, for instance), could combat the hormonal assault on hair follicles.

Doctors and patients discovered that Proscar, originally prescribed to treat benign prostate enlargement, had an exciting, positive side effect: It grew hair on bald men's heads—"regular" (called *terminal*) hair, not peach fuzz. The stage was finally set for a truly effective balding treatment.

To understand why this is the case, here's a crash course on how testosterone causes hair loss: For many years, the scientific community and the rest of us were under the impression that androgenetic alopecia (male pattern baldness) was caused by the predominance of the male sex hormone, testosterone. While testosterone does play a role in the balding process, the accumulation of scientific study over the course of decades has revealed that dihydrotestosterone (DHT), a derivative of testosterone, is actually the main culprit.

Testosterone converts to DHT with the aid of the enzyme Type II 5-alpha-reductase, which is held in a hair follicle's oil glands. Scientists now believe that it is not the amount of circulating testosterone but the *level of DHT* binding to receptors in scalp follicles that determines hair loss. DHT shrinks hair follicles, making it impossible for healthy hair to survive.

The first evidence of the relationship between male pattern baldness and testosterone was discovered by a psychiatrist early in the twentieth century. At the time, castration was commonly performed on some of the more uncontrollable psychiatric patients in sanatoriums. Castrating these patients not only eliminated their sex drive, it also produced a calming effect, much like a sedative.

This particular doctor noted that one of his castrated patients had a full head of hair, while the patient's uninstitutionalized twin brother who came to visit was very bald. The doctor then noted that the mentally ill twin had been castrated *before* the onset of puberty. The doctor was curious: If a pure form of testosterone was injected into the castrated twin, would it affect his full head of hair? Within weeks of the injection, the twin began to lose his hair.

In 1942 James B. Hamilton of Yale published a report in the *American Journal of Anatomy* detailing his studies of men whose testes had been removed before puberty for medical reasons and noting the fact that these men never went bald, even if they had bald relatives. When these castrated men were given testosterone injections, however, their hair began to fall out, and they were soon almost as bald as some of their relatives. If the testosterone injections stopped, their hair loss stopped progressing. Interestingly, if the men came from families with few bald men, the testosterone injections didn't cause much baldness. This was the first time science had noted that baldness was linked to both hormones and genes.

These studies revealed that if testosterone has never been introduced into the hormonal pool, then hair loss will not occur. But once testosterone is activated (at puberty, for those who have not had the misfortune of being castrated), it creates a biochemical reaction in people who have a genetic predisposition to androgenetic alopecia, male pattern baldness.

In the case of the twin at the sanatorium who grew bald once testosterone was introduced into his body, it's important to note that when the doctor stopped giving him testosterone, the twin did regrow some of his hair, but not all of it, since many of his hair follicles had died.

Only decades later would scientists discover that follicles die not from the testosterone itself but from its follicle-killing derivative, DHT, and that hair will not grow from dead follicles.

The drug finasteride was the result of a long-term research project at Merck that began initially in the mid-1950s, according to the company. At that time, Merck scientists were conducting research into the role of androgens (like DHT) in benign prostate enlargement and male pattern baldness. By the 1960s, Merck researchers had learned that Type II 5-alpha-reductase (an enzyme) was necessary to complete the conversion of testosterone to DHT, and this was the basis for the development of finasteride, which inhibits this particular enzyme.

Merck decided to focus first on prostate enlargement, the company says, because the medical need for a treatment of the condition was greater.

The 1970s brought more confirmation of the DHT and Type II 5-alpha-reductase connection to male pattern baldness. Scientists in the Dominican Republic were looking at the cases of male children who, though born with XY chromosomes, grew up looking like females. Only when they went through puberty was it apparent that they were male. Their genitalia were almost nonexistent as children, but they then grew to normal size once the body manufactured testosterone at the onset of puberty.

The researchers noted that these boys never lost their hair as they grew older. Although all of these boys had normal—and in some cases raised—levels of male hormones, they all had *no trace of Type II 5-alpha-reductase,* the enzyme that converts testosterone to DHT, which then kills hair follicles in the male pattern baldness areas of the scalp.

In the mid-1980s, Merck scientists working with their prostate drug finasteride, marketed as Proscar, knew that cases of male pattern baldness were rare in men with low levels of Type II 5-alpha-reductase. The company then turned its attention to using finasteride to treat male pattern baldness. They would need separate FDA approval to market finasteride as a hair-loss drug treatment, though, so in 1992 Merck began testing the drug (which they would eventually market under the brand name Propecia) specifically to treat male pattern baldness so they could head down the road to FDA approval.

Remember that it's actually in the hair follicles that testosterone converts to the more powerful DHT, which behaves differently depending upon where on the body those follicles are located. The male pattern baldness areas of the head—the front, temples, and crown—are more sensitive to testosterone and therefore quicker to convert it to DHT. As DHT shrinks a hair follicle, shortening a hair's growth cycle, a normal hair's diameter lessens and lessens over time until the hair is tiny and fine. Ultimately, no hair can grow when the follicle dies.

Elsewhere on the body, DHT behaves differently. It actually *stimulates* hair growth in follicles located on the chest, back, shoulders, eyebrows, and ears, even though it kills hair follicles on the scalp.

Geographical and cultural influences also affect hormones. Compared to Asian men, Americans have more of the enzyme that converts testosterone to DHT and thus have more body hair and more baldness. The role that a culture's food choices may play in the action of our hormones is the subject of ongoing study by scientists (and is discussed in Chapter Two).

Women naturally have far less testosterone than men—actually just a trace of the hormone. But when a woman has more than the usual amount in her system—because of medication, a hormone-producing growth, or another problem—she can also develop male pattern baldness. Because finasteride can cause birth defects in a male fetus, women of childbearing age who are not sterile should not take finasteride. Although it is not intended for use by women, in certain circumstances a doctor may prescribe it for a woman with androgenetic alopecia.

Apparently baldness leads to more baldness. In balding areas, the oil glands in the hair follicle become larger. Since it's these glands that hold the enzyme that converts testosterone to the follicle-killing DHT, there's always a lot of the enzyme in these enlarged glands in balding areas, ready to further weaken the follicles. Oil gland activity is also increased by higher amounts of circulating hormones.

Hormones are not static. Testosterone levels in some men drop by 10 percent each decade after age thirty. Testosterone levels peak in the fall and are lowest in the spring. During the spring low, hair grows the most. As testosterone levels rise, heading toward fall, so does hair loss. By fall, twice as much hair is lost than was lost in the spring. Both men and women have a similar hair growth seasonal cycle. The cyclic nature of both our hair and hormones is one reason why hair loss can increase in the short term even when you are experiencing a long-term slowdown of hair loss (and a long-term increase in hair growth) while on a treatment that controls baldness.

Male pattern baldness is also genetic, and the gene is passed to a child from either parent, *not* just the mother, as had been previously thought.

Finasteride in Action

When I discovered that Merck was studying their prostate drug Proscar (finasteride) for its

13

baldness prevention and treatment potential, the 1 mg. dose of the drug they would name Propecia was in the second phase of its FDA study. It was 1994, and with the third-phase human trials for efficacy still to come, FDA approval for finasteride's use as Propecia, a drug to prevent and treat hair loss, would be years away.

Although minoxidil had bought me some time (about two years), I was not the best candidate for the drug, so I needed to explore other options, including finasteride, as soon as possible.

I wanted to take finasteride *now*. But until its approval by the FDA specifically for hair loss, men could only get the drug marketed as Proscar, a 5 mg. pill, for prostate treatment. And if a man didn't have any prostate trouble, he'd have to convince a doctor to prescribe Proscar for him anyway.

I called my hair specialist very excitedly and asked him if he knew about Proscar and its hair-saving side effect. He said that he knew about the drug. When I asked what he thought about it, he told me that if I took the drug at my age (I was almost twenty-nine), I would likely become impotent and eventually take on female characteristics, such as breast enlargement and curvaceous hips. (I discovered later that many physicians were under this misconception and were causing unnecessary worry. It wasn't Proscar but a previous generation of prostate drugs that had these unfortunate "feminizing" side effects among many of the men who took them.) He affirmed that he provided the only safe and effective antibaldness treatment in the world and that I should stick to his concoction.

Since I enjoyed sex and had no desire to develop a girlish figure, I took his advice. I stuck to his treatment for a few more months. I was still losing my hair. I began to notice that when I went to his office to get my supply of "product" at $90 a pop, there was more and more anti–Proscar literature in his waiting room, photocopied sheets noting only its adverse side effects.

I read some of these and noticed that all of the men who were studied in the original Proscar FDA trials for approval as a prostate drug were over the age of forty. *All* had enlarged prostates. Chances are that many of them suffered from impotence for reasons having nothing to do with Proscar.

These photocopied sheets listed the possible side effects, and there were *only five,* including possible lowering of libido, partial impotence, and smaller volume of ejaculant. In about 60 percent of the very few men with these side effects, these symptoms were transient and went away during the course of treatment. (Also, the 5 mg. Proscar pill used in these studies contained five times the amount of finasteride Merck planned to use in its

15

1 mg. Propecia pill for the treatment of baldness.) Nothing about the side effects of Proscar mentioned anything about turning into a woman.

The doctor was definitely threatened by the possibility that people could save their hair by popping a pill for far less than the cost of his virtually useless concoction. I stopped using his product and started to research Proscar.

Finasteride is a synthetic compound that specifically inhibits Type II 5-alpha-reductase, the enzyme that converts testosterone into a more potent androgen dihydrotestosterone (DHT). Finasteride, when marketed as a 1 mg. pill to treat baldness under the brand name Propecia, can decrease DHT concentrations by approximately 60 percent (Proscar's 5 mg. dose decreases DHT by 70 percent).

Contrary to what my hair specialist told me, I discovered that research has shown that in patients being treated with a 5 mg. dose of Proscar during a 12-week period, the hypothalamic-pituitary-testicular axis was not affected. In other words, if the patient reacted normally to the drug, he experienced no adverse sexual side effects. Because a balding man now regaining his hair was likely to feel better about his appearance, men taking finasteride might even experience an increase in their libido.

The possibility of experiencing any of the five possible side effects was rare. The antidepressant that my hair specialist wanted me to take (he apparently thought that those not happy about losing their hair should cheer up about it) has *sixty-one* possible adverse side effects including impotence, ejaculation problems, abnormal bleeding, and, ironically, *hair loss.* More than 15 percent of the patients treated with this antidepressant drug experienced these adverse side effects. Only 3.7 percent of those taking the 5 mg. Proscar pill experienced any side effects—and sixty percent of those 3.7 percent experienced the side effects only temporarily, and in time they subsided completely. Aspirin has more documented adverse side effects than Proscar. Aspirin's list of side effects includes nausea, loss of blood in the stool, stomach ulcers and bleeding, hives, liver damage, and visual difficulties.

I couldn't understand why so many medical professionals were so anti–Proscar. Their propaganda also raised the fear of possible birth defects in male fetuses if finasteride was passed through sperm, but according to the research the chances of that were practically nil. And a man could always temporarily stop using the drug if he were inclined to impregnate someone, or he could wear a condom to help prevent pregnancy. Women can also rely on their array of birth control methods to prevent pregnancy if their partner is taking finasteride.

The bottom line is that these hair specialists knew that a drug as affordable, effective, and low risk as Proscar would take some of the lining out of their pockets. It wouldn't be the first time that professionals in health care—or any other industry—would be resistant to advances that would jeopardize the economic status quo.

I wanted to start treatment with Proscar. I was not about to let someone else control my destiny. I wanted to keep my hair, and I was willing to do anything that I felt was safe.

I called every hair specialist in the nation, trying to get a prescription for Proscar, and almost everyone thought that I was out of my mind. One well-known hair specialist in New York did say that he was supplying some of his patients with the drug. He told me that he had seen some very impressive results. The catch was that he'd only allow his patients to use it in conjunction with his minoxidil concoction. I only wanted the Proscar. But he wouldn't provide it for me unless I used it *his* way, which would cost around $200 per month for the Proscar pill–minoxidil topical lotion package.

Finally, I asked a physician friend what he thought about prescribing Proscar for male pattern baldness. He looked it up in his *Physician's Desk Reference* and said that it was worth trying as long as I had some blood tests done and was willing to be tested a few times a year. I agreed, and he gave me a prescription for Proscar.

As one of the very few men outside of Merck's FDA studies to take finasteride to treat hair loss, I felt like some kind of pioneer when I popped that first pill in December 1994. I had a very strong feeling that this was going to help me, and I knew that when it did I would share this information, as well as everything else I was learning about hair loss, with anyone and everyone who needed it.

By early 1995, within two months of starting Proscar, my excessive hair fall-out had ceased. I had no adverse side effects, sexual or otherwise. I had been literally counting hairs and saving them in plastic bags and labeling them to compare weekly counts (C'mon, we've all been there, right?), so I was very aware of what was happening on my head. Before the third month began, the hair count had not only stabilized—I only lost a little each day, just like someone who *isn't* balding—but hair was growing back, too.

The hair on the sides of my head had become very thin over the years, and I had some recession as well. That hair had now begun to grow back.

Within twelve months, ninety-five percent of my hair was actually growing again. It was still a little thinner than it had been before the onset of male pattern baldness, but I was no longer concerned with losing my hair and the unwanted change in my appearance.

My male pattern baldness had not progressed since I began taking finasteride.

In August 1996, I started the Web site "Major Hair Loss News" (http://members.aol.com/hairman96) in order to share reliable information about the biology of hair loss, treatment options, and other information that consumers may need to stay informed and to protect themselves when dealing with the unregulated hair-loss industry.

The response to the Web site has been both overwhelming and gratifying: During the first year alone, nearly 10,000 men and women contacted me for help, and I supplied them with an information package that included details on finasteride, diet, herbal treatments, hair-transplant surgery, an update on physicians, and other research and practical information, charging only $5.95 to cover printing and postage. I soon realized that this Web site was giving real hope to people who had all but thrown in the towel. I have received calls, letters, and E-mail from people all over the world, and I consult with leading hair-loss experts and researchers.

What began as a personal quest ended up as my life's work: consumer advocacy for the "hair impaired."

I knew what they had been through and were still dealing with. I had been there myself.

Randy from Kansas wrote: "The information that you provided regarding DHT and the substances that can counter it was the first substantive data I've ever received on hair loss and hair growth. I've got to believe that countless other guys around the country, even the world, would benefit greatly from what you have to offer."

I was determined to see to it that those battling hair loss wouldn't have to have that problem compounded by unreliable information, greedy marketers of useless products and damaging procedures, and other abuses.

"My brother is twenty-four years old and has full receding baldness. He is extremely handsome regardless, and yet he has been covering his head with a cap for more than three years," wrote one woman in an E-mail that is representative of the pain and frustration of thousands of others with whom I've been in contact. "He feels so terrible, he doesn't feel like looking at anyone and barely keeps his job because he prefers to miss meetings—so many people would see his head. We love him, but he tries to evade facial contact. I love him, hair or not. I am worried and sad. I've heard on the Net that you have helped a great many people. Can you please help my brother, he is really suffering. I've been in contact with hundreds of men and women who say that the treatments you recommend are the only thing that's helped them. Please help my brother."

I can identify with the pain every time I read a plea like that. I was relieved that I had helped myself, and in turn had been able to help others, but when some of the E-mails and letters began referring to me as the "Hair Messiah," and when the praise for my information and efforts began pouring in along with reports of success with the treatments I'd recommended, I felt a bit strange.

Andres from Argentina wrote: "I am taking finasteride and I am seeing very encouraging results. I think that what you are doing is very important for people who suffer from this problem."

Ken wrote that he hoped my work would "revolutionize the hair industry and take out all the scams and quacks."

Tony kept me posted about his battle with hair loss. After receiving my information package, which included information on finasteride, he said, "I immediately called my doctor. Luckily, she had been my physician for many years, because at first she was rather hesitant to give me a prescription. After thumbing through her [drug] book, she decided that it probably wouldn't hurt to give it a try. She prescribed 5 mg. Proscar with the stipulation that I return for checkups. I am happy to report that I have had NO side effects or adverse reactions as a result of taking Proscar. This sounds kind of over the top, but I would have to say that life has really changed for me. In the past, because of my hair loss, time was my enemy. Every day marked the gradual decline in my looks. As a result of Proscar, I now look forward to the next day, and the day after. After three months I already noticed hair regrowth. The word tomorrow has a much more promising ring to it."

Kevin wrote: "Knowing you're losing your hair is frustrating and heartbreaking. Especially for me because I'm only twenty-three. I noticed my loss when I was about twenty and I thought that there was no way this could be happening to me this young. I used to have nice, thick, wavy hair that I used to think was troublesome. I wish I still had hair like I did back then. I guess you really don't appreciate what you're blessed with until it gradually disappears. Being so young, and still in college, looks are important to me. Unfortunately, I believe my hair loss is affecting my looks and it hurts me very much. I probably wouldn't care if I was sixty years old, but I'm only one-third of that age. I think I've spent way too much time worrying about my condition."

Letters and E-mails like these continue to pour in. You'll read about more of these in our discussion of herbal treatments in Chapter Three.

But before we continue with finasteride's road

to FDA approval for marketing as Propecia, here's the story of Brian, whose own road led him to finasteride and herbal treatments after he'd seen my Web site.

"After reading the information you sent me, I wondered how you dealt with the stress over all those years of trying everything. It can really get to you. Now that I'm taking Proscar I have *hope,*" he wrote. "My story started about nine years ago. I know this because I found an old prescription bottle of lotion from my dermatologist. My hair was very slowly thinning, so slowly that I didn't notice it too much."

Brian's doctor had given him this lotion to help treat the tingling and itching he often felt as his hair loss gradually progressed. Of course, it did nothing to stop the hair loss.

"About a year and a half ago, I noticed it looked a little thinner again and I decided to try Rogaine. It was over-the-counter now, so what the heck. Seven months later, it hadn't done much of anything at all for me. I stopped the Rogaine," he continued. "Then my seven-year-old daughter was sitting across the living room from me and said, 'I can see right through your head.' I knew what she meant. If I sit in the car and look in the rear-view mirror, looking at the front of my head, I can see light through the back! I stood in front of the mirror one day and put another mirror in the back of my head. What I saw was the typical upside-down horseshoe baldness pattern starting. The only way I can describe that kind of shock is to imagine being asleep in the middle of the night and waking up and seeing a stranger standing at the foot of your bed. Kind of like watching a horror movie or something. The shock just hits you. You start to notice people talking to *you,* but looking at your *head.*"

After learning about finasteride, Brian went back to his dermatologist.

"I asked him what kind of treatments were new since I first saw him years ago, and he said I could try Rogaine. I told him, 'That won't work for me and my level of hair loss. How about Proscar?' He said he would be going to a conference in the fall and would let me know what he thought after that. But what if I waited that few months and then he *still* wouldn't let me try it? Then I've wasted a few more months. Doctors don't look at this as a real medical problem. They shrug it off. That is, of course, the ones who aren't making money off of it. I recently got an E-mail from one of the Rogaine/Retin-A doctors. He strongly suggests not using Proscar. Of course he does. He's trying to sell *his* product. So many people just take this problem for granted and just accept it. I don't accept things easily. I am amazed at all the sites on the Internet that sell hair-promoting shampoos, vitamins, herbal liquids, and they aren't cheap. I've used some really bad-smelling brown herbal liquid stuff on my head that came in a small, cheap, plastic bottle with a label glued to it made on a copy machine. I've paid for information telling me about Thymu-Skin. I've seen videos advertised on the Internet for two hundred bucks that will teach you how to massage your head back to healthy hair. Of course, in my search, I read a lot about 5-alpha-reductase and DHT, and so I started to research this more because it made sense. I finally came to your Web site, which was describing what I was going through. After getting all of your information, and talking to you on the phone, I realized that I had found someone out there who *really* wants to help."

Now taking finasteride and herbs, Brian is experiencing less hair fall-out and gradual hair regrowth.

Propecia's Road to FDA Approval

On December 19, 1996, Merck & Co. filed with the FDA for approval the results of their third-phase study of their hair-loss drug Propecia (1 mg. finasteride).

Three months later, on March 23, 1997, they

presented data from these phase-three (human trials) studies to the American Academy of Dermatology meeting in San Francisco.

The protocol for all of the studies within these human trials included the following:

- A total of 1,879 men participated.
- The men ranged in age from eighteen to forty-one, and they participated at a number of centers in the United States and worldwide.
- For twelve months each man daily received either a 1 mg. oral dose of Propecia or a placebo.
- The studies were double-blind, meaning that neither the patient nor the clinician administering the dose knew whether the patient was receiving Propecia or the placebo.
- Improvement was assessed by research investigators who examined each patient, by an expert panel of dermatologists who reviewed patient photos, and by the patients themselves, who filled out questionnaires at each visit.
- Each of the men participating had mild to moderate, but not complete, hair loss.
- Safety was evaluated through clinical and laboratory monitoring and analysis, and an analysis of adverse events.

The data presented at this March meeting was from studies of 1,553 men with predominant thinning of hair in the vertex area (top of the head). Overall improvement was seen as early as three months, with continued improvement over the course of the twelve-month trial period. After twelve months, the results from the vertex studies were as follows:

- 86 percent of the men taking Propecia maintained or showed an increase in the amount of hair based on hair counts during the course of the studies, compared to 42 percent of the men receiving the placebo.
- 14 percent of the men taking Propecia lost hair (measuring any decrease in hair count from the baseline established at the start of the study), while 58 percent of the men in the placebo group continued to lose hair.

The difference between the men taking Propecia and the men taking the placebo is most dramatic in these two sets of results because they are based on actual hair counts, the most objective form of result assessment.

- Clinical investigators rated 65 percent of men treated with Propecia as having substantial increased hair growth, compared to 37 percent of the men taking the placebo.

- An expert panel of dermatologists evaluating patient photos rated 48 percent of patients treated with Propecia as having increased hair growth, while only 7 percent of patients taking the placebo were reported to show improvement.
- In the patient questionnaires, 68 percent of men taking Propecia reported that their hair loss had slowed, compared to 45 percent of those taking the placebo. Improvement was noted as early as the third month, when those percentages were 54 and 44 respectively.

"The clinical relevance of the increased hair growth measured by hair counts was substantiated by the significant improvements perceived by patients and through complementary measures such as the investigator and expert panel assessments," said Keith Kaufman, M.D., director of clinical research at Merck & Co., based in Rahway, New Jersey.

Three months later, on June 17, 1997, Merck presented data to the World Congress of Dermatology, meeting in Sydney, Australia, this time from their phase-three human trials studies of 326 men with frontal hair thinning.

As in the vertex studies, men with frontal thinning also benefited from Propecia, which prevented further hair loss and increased hair growth.

- Clinical investigators rated 52 percent of men treated with Propecia as having substantial hair growth, compared to 31 percent of men treated with the placebo.
- An expert panel of dermatologists evaluating patient photos rated 37 percent of patients treated with Propecia as having increased hair growth, while only 7 percent of patients taking the placebo were reported to show improvement.
- In the patient questionnaires, 53 percent of men taking Propecia reported an improvement in the appearance of their hair, while 30 percent of the men taking the placebo reported improvement. In addition, 65 percent of men taking Propecia, compared to 45 percent of men taking the placebo, reported that their hair loss had slowed.

Slightly lower effectiveness rates in the frontal studies are due to the fact that frontal hair is generally harder to regrow than hair at the vertex.

Investigators also reported a significant improvement for men treated with Propecia compared to those taking the placebo in hair density and pattern in three sections of the scalp—frontal, mid area, and vertex—throughout the studies. Regarding the data reported in the frontal study, Merck's Keith Kaufman, M.D., said, "The frontal study is unique because hair-loss studies in men typically evaluate hair growth at the vertex. Frontal thinning is commonly seen in men, and it is what they may first notice when they look in the mirror."

SIDE EFFECTS

Finasteride lowers the numbers in the PSA test (the prostate cancer screening test given as part of your general physical exam), and may therefore give you a false low-numbered status, thus masking levels of Prostate Specific Antigen that are actually higher. Tell your doctor if you are taking finasteride so that he will be able to properly interpret your PSA tests and order other screening tests that are not affected by the use of finasteride.

Regarding side effects, Merck's phase three studies of all the men participating show that "for the overwhelming majority of the men—96 percent—these side effects were not reported," said Dr. Kaufman.

When side effects did occur, they "were reversible in men who discontinued therapy, and

even resolved in many of these patients who pre-
ferred to continue treatment," Dr. Kaufman noted.

No birth defects were reported when several
patients who were using finasteride impregnated
someone.

The tolerability of Propecia was reinforced by
the data from these human trials. The drug was
very well tolerated, with most patients reporting
no significant side effects. The overall safety pro-
file for Propecia and the placebo was similar. Side
effects were infrequent and occurred in a small
number of men. The only side effects occurring in
more than 1 percent of patients were the following:

- Decreased libido: 1.8 percent of men treated
  with Propecia vs. 1.3 percent on placebo.
- Erectile dysfunction: 1.3 percent of men
  treated with Propecia vs. 0.7 percent on placebo.
- Decreased volume of ejaculate: 0.8 percent
  of men treated with Propecia vs. 0.4 percent
  on placebo.
- Discontinuation of therapy due to adverse
  side effects occurred in 1.7 percent of 945
  men on Propecia and 2.1 percent of 934 men
  on a placebo.

Propecia is for use by men only. Women "who
are or may be pregnant must not use Propecia,

since it may cause a specific birth defect in a male fetus," warned the company.

In their report of these FDA trial studies, Merck explained that "Propecia works by treating an underlying cause of male pattern hair loss by inhibiting the production of DHT, which is believed to be a major cause of hair loss. The enzyme Type II 5-alpha-reductase is involved in the production of DHT. Propecia inhibits the action of Type II 5-alpha-reductase, thereby decreasing DHT concentrations in treated men by approximately 60 percent."

Although male pattern baldness is genetically linked, its onset is triggered by the presence of DHT in the hair follicles of susceptible scalp areas, so "the ability to increase hair growth and prevent further hair loss by specifically lowering DHT with finasteride 1 mg. provides a potential new oral therapeutic option with an excellent risk-benefit ratio for the treatment of men with male pattern hair loss," Dr. Kaufman noted in Merck's report of their data. "This approach represents an important advance in our understanding of the science of hair loss. An important step in the development of Propecia was understanding the biology of male pattern hair loss and DHT's role in it. This knowledge has led to a new paradigm in treating men with this condition."

The positive results I have experienced while

taking finasteride were confirmed by Merck's studies.

Merck submitted their application and study results to the FDA for clearance to market finasteride in 1 mg. pills under the brand name Propecia as the first oral treatment taken once a day for the prevention of further hair loss and for regrowth in the most common sites of hair thinning in men.

On December 22, 1997, the FDA approved Merck's application to market Propecia, and the prescription drug was shipped to pharmacies only weeks later, in January 1998.

With the introduction of Propecia and the many drugs that are sure to jump on the hair-loss treatment bandwagon in the coming years, treating male pattern baldness will be like treating any other chronic manageable disorder, such as hypertension or diabetes. Once the onset of the disorder makes itself apparent, the patient can go to the doctor and get a prescription for the problem.

Propecia can be used alone or in conjunction with herbs and/or a specific nutritional program that enhances hair retention and regrowth. Propecia is also a very effective adjunct treatment to hair-replacement surgery.

Baldness treatment pioneer O'Tar Norwood, M.D., who set the standard of pattern hair-loss classification with the Norwood Scale, has been following the ongoing hair-loss research and, like many other specialists, shares in the enthusiasm surrounding the breakthrough that finasteride represents with its ability to combat DHT's major role in male pattern baldness.

"The fact that it slows down hair loss," Dr. Norwood says, "is revolutionary. I especially encourage young patients who are too early for transplant surgery to use it, as well as those who can use it as an adjunct to hair-transplant surgery."

Those men with mild to moderate baldness will benefit. For those with more extensive baldness, the drug will reduce further hair loss and will encourage hair regrowth in those follicles that are still alive.

Propecia may be used alone or as an adjunct to other treatments, including nutritional, herbal, and surgical. Although Merck's studies are quite reassuring regarding the extremely low incidences of side effects, and the temporary nature of those side effects, caution should always be used when determining if any drug is right for *you*.

William R. Rassman, M.D., a leading hair specialist who with his colleague Robert M. Bernstein, M.D., perfected the follicular hair-transplant technique in the United States, believes that Propecia can be used alone or as an adjunct to other treatments, including hair-transplantation surgery, but he reminds us that as with many drugs, even those that have been used for a number of years, "all the long-term risks may not be known yet."

Now that the first treatment that actually acts upon the cause of male pattern baldness is on the market, men have the opportunity, if they so choose, to incorporate this drug into their hair-loss prevention and treatment.

2

THE HORMONAL EFFECTS
OF DIET ON HAIR LOSS

Your remedies shall be your food, and
your food shall be your remedies.
—HIPPOCRATES

Food plays a profound role in the effectiveness of
drug and herbal therapy when treating any condition, including hair loss. By utilizing food for its
medicinal, healing, and system-altering properties, you can also control your hormone levels, including the levels of DHT, the main culprit in male
pattern baldness, and therefore further control
your hair loss.

I have been able to do just that: use a specific
kind of diet that boosts the efficacy of the drug
Propecia (finasteride) and herbs that control hair

loss, and that helps keep certain hormones from adversely affecting my hair.

In this chapter you will learn how hormones can be regulated by diet, how scientists have found crucial links between foods, health, and hair loss, and how you can easily follow a hair-supporting way of eating that also protects your heart and overall health and fitness.

How Hormones Control Your Body

When we think of hormones, we usually think of testosterone and estrogen, the two major human sex hormones. These hormones not only regulate our sexual characteristics, reproductive system, and sexual appetites, they are also vital in maintaining our overall good health.

But hormones of *all* kinds regulate *every* working mechanism in the body. They regulate the simplest to the most intricate bodily functions. They regulate our emotions too: love, fear, anxiety, stress, joy, and everything in between.

The body facilitates communication among cells in two ways: One is by electrical impulses that travel through nerve fibers called neurons, and the other is by chemicals that are carried through the endocrine system. It's this second, chemical system that uses hormones as messengers.

The speed of electrical message transmission through neurons is more than lightning quick, it's virtually instantaneous. The brain tells the leg to move, and in that instant the leg moves.

The endocrine system, however, communicates in a more leisurely manner. The glands in this chemical system release hormones into the bloodstream, which carries them to all parts of the body. It takes anywhere from a few minutes to several hours for these hormones to reach their destinations.

The glands in the endocrine system are located throughout the body:

- The *pituitary gland* is just beneath the base of the front part of the brain.
- The *thyroid* and *parathyroid glands* are at the front of the neck, just above the top of the breastbone.
- The *adrenal glands* sit adjacent to the top of the kidneys, one gland above each kidney.
- The *pancreas* is behind the stomach in the abdominal cavity.
- The *ovaries* (in women only) are in the pelvic area, just below the navel.
- The *testes* (in men only) are nestled in the

scrotum, the external pouch behind the penis.

Hormones are very powerful, even in the smallest amounts, and they are released in one of the body's many exquisitely timed and balanced systems. The *hypothalamus,* a control center in the brain about the size of a macadamia nut, regulates the body's basic functions, including sleeping, eating, and reproduction. One of its vital duties is to control the endocrine system by controlling the pituitary gland, whose job is to receive messages about an organ's or other area's need for a particular hormone and then to either secrete that hormone itself or secrete a substance that causes another gland in the endocrine system to make and release the desired hormone.

The hormones from a man's testes, as well as those from his adrenal glands, are responsible for all manner of things "male," from male physical and sexual characteristics to sexual and reproductive function. The testes produce the male sex hormone testosterone, and, as you'll remember, testosterone converts to dihydrotestosterone (DHT) with the help of the enzyme 5-alpha-reductase. It's the DHT that shrinks hair follicles in men with the gene for male pattern baldness, leading ultimately to the death of hair follicles and therefore hair loss. Forms of the generic drug finasteride (Proscar and Propecia), as well as herbs you'll read about in Chapter Three, inhibit the body's production of the 5-alpha-reductase enzyme, thus significantly reducing the body's levels of the hair-follicle-killing DHT. What we eat also affects testosterone and DHT levels, so it is also possible to curb hair loss by choosing foods for their medicinal properties and avoiding other foods because of their role in the hormonal chain of events that can lead to hair loss.

The testes also produce androgens, hormones that, like testosterone, stimulate the development of male secondary sex characteristics from puberty onward, such as growth of the penis, growth of body hair, deepening of the voice, and increased muscle mass. Androgens are classified as corticosteroids, and they are produced not only by the testes but by the adrenal glands as well.

The Sugar Connection to Hair Loss

The pancreas also comes into play in our discussion of hormones, diet, and hair loss because of its crucial role in regulating the body's sugar levels. Before you can understand the connection, though, you have to understand how the pancreas works, which you may know something about if you or someone you know has diabetes.

The pancreas creates *insulin* and *glucagon,* which both maintain stable blood-sugar levels. Insulin helps your body's cells use glucose (a sugar) for fuel, thereby lowering the amount of sugar remaining in the bloodstream. Glucagon stimulates the liver to release its stored sugar into the blood when the amount of sugar in the bloodstream needs to be raised. These two hormones play off each other to keep your blood-sugar levels in a balanced state.

When the pancreas can't produce enough insulin or the body can't use the insulin the pancreas makes, diabetes, a condition characterized by a chronically high level of blood sugar, is the result. This means that the sugar isn't able to go from the bloodstream to the cells where it's vitally needed to fuel the body, or to the liver, where it's stored until needed for fuel.

In the opposite situation—known as hypoglycemia or low blood sugar—the body's sugar is used for fuel by the cells to such an extent that not enough circulates in the bloodstream. This can be caused by something as simple as not eating often enough for blood-sugar levels to be replenished (that's the light-headed or queasy feeling you get if you haven't eaten in a few hours or all day) or from an excess of insulin.

There is a crucial link between your body's insulin level and its testosterone level, and by controlling the former you can also control the latter. This is an important element in preventing hair loss and creating an internal physiological environment conducive to hair growth, as you will see later in this chapter.

Preventing Hair Loss with a Low-Fat, Sugar-Balancing Diet

As noted earlier, you can use food as a drug, in a very real sense, in order to regulate your hormones and therefore control hair loss.

Foods affect hormones very quickly, usually within just a few weeks. Scientists know that diets high in animal fats trigger your body to release more testosterone into your bloodstream. Studies show that people on low-fat or vegetarian diets have lower levels of testosterone in their blood. A high-fat diet also increases estrogen in both men and women. Someone who is overweight is also more likely to have a higher level of estrogen, and doctors believe that is why obese men can experience breast enlargement. In general, then, a high-fat diet throws your body's normal hormonal balance completely out of whack.

This, of course, directly affects hair loss, since testosterone plays such a crucial role in male pattern baldness. Studies have also shown that a high-fat diet reduces the amount of a protein known as *sex hormone binding globulin.* This protein keeps a sex hormone inactive until it's needed by the body. With less of this protein in your bloodstream, more testosterone circulates, ready to be converted to DHT at the hair follicle if conditions there are favorable. Oil glands in the hair follicle hold 5-alpha-reductase, the enzyme that converts testosterone into DHT, and higher amounts of circulating hormones, including testosterone, can increase this oil gland activity. To make matters worse, in balding areas the oil glands in the hair follicle are larger than the oil glands in the areas of your scalp that are not balding.

In an oft-cited 1985 study, Japanese researcher Masumi Inaba published a report showing this phenomenon in action. He noted that there had been an increase in the incidence of balding among Japanese men that coincided with the increasing Westernization of their food habits: They were eating more red meat, thus introducing far more animal fat into their diets than had Japanese men in previous generations. Inaba theorized that this increased intake of animal fat directly led to the increase of the incidence of balding because the higher levels of animal fat cause the oil glands in the hair follicles to grow, leading to more DHT production and therefore more damage to the follicles.

In my search for the most effective hormonal diet, I read countless studies, articles, and books, including *The Zone,* the 1995 bestseller by Barry Sears, Ph.D. In *The Zone,* I found more clues to the food balance that hormonally supports hair growth and fights hair loss.

Dr. Sears, a biochemist, was directly involved in creating the delivery system for several cancer drugs, including AZT, one of the drugs used to treat AIDS. In 1982 Dr. Sears was working in the world of lipid research, which includes the behavior of hormones. That year, the Nobel Prize for physiology and medicine was awarded to Sune Bergstorm and Bengt Samuelsson of the Karolinska Institute in Stockholm, and John Vane of the Royal College of Surgeons in England, for research on a powerful class of hormones called *eicosanoids* (pronounced eye-KAH-sah-noids).

Eicosanoids are among the most powerful and important substances in the body. Dr. Sears calls them "the molecular glue" that holds the body together, the master switches that control *all* human bodily functions, and as such they control every system, including the systems that govern how much fat we store in our bodies, a key factor in testosterone behavior.

Dr. Sears realized that if you can control these hormones, you can control virtually every aspect of human physiology. Although baldness was not mentioned in the book, after reading *The Zone,* I deduced that it just might be possible to use a low-animal-fat, sugar-balancing diet similar to *The Zone's*—whose effects control testosterone, insulin, and eicosanoids—to combat hair loss by creating an internal environment of more favorable hormonal balance and therefore lower DHT levels. That would make it even easier for the body to respond to the drug finasteride (Proscar/Propecia).

At that point, I seemed to have reached a hair regrowth plateau. The progression of my hair loss had ceased, but so had the significant hair regrowth that I had been experiencing during the first year and a half while taking finasteride.

After just two months on a sugar-balancing diet, I began to see substantial changes in my body and, just as important, on my head. Not only was I performing better in everyday life—and getting trimmer—but, to my delight, I was growing more hair back. I had been correct in assuming that I would be able to boost the efficacy of finasteride by keeping my hormones in check. I also continued to have *no* adverse side effects from the drug treatment.

I contacted the offices of Dr. Sears to inform

him of my experiences. He had received several calls inquiring about whether a sugar-balancing diet might help fight hair loss, so his office began referring those calls to me. I told all who called about my positive experiences using a sugar-balancing diet to fight hair loss, and I also discussed finasteride and herbal therapies with them. A large majority of those to whom I recommended this diet-and-herbal combination experienced significant positive results, including hair regrowth.

After a few months, I informed Dr. Sears's office that I was working on a book about hair loss, which would include controlling the effects of DHT as it pertains to male pattern baldness.

Dr. Sears called me the next day, and we discussed my experiences, information gathering, and consumer advocacy. After talking about the significance that a sugar-balancing diet (like *The Zone* diet or one followed by diabetic patients) played in the efficacy of treatment for male pattern baldness, in my experience and that of the many men I recommended it to, Dr. Sears was intrigued by my discovery and agreed with my findings. He later explained to me how the hormonal effects of a sugar-balancing diet, which go beyond just testosterone, could indeed be a blessing to balding men.

"At the molecular level, balding can be viewed as a hormonal disturbance condition," Dr. Sears said. "It is clear that the hormone dihydrotestosterone (DHT), which is a breakdown product of testosterone, is a major contributor to baldness; therefore, interventions that lower DHT levels should have a beneficial effect on balding. The drug known as Proscar (finasteride) is one such agent. It inhibits the enzyme that converts testosterone into DHT. This is why Proscar is the primary drug used for the treatment of enlarged prostates. Another biochemical approach is modulating the production of testosterone itself, which can be accomplished using dietary measures."

Dr. Sears then went on to explain how a low-fat, sugar-balancing diet does this, and how insulin, another vital hormone, plays a pivotal role.

This kind of diet is "based on keeping another hormone, insulin, in a tight zone: not too high, not too low. By doing so, one is able to control the body's production of an essential fatty acid called arachidonic acid. By controlling the levels of arachidonic acid, the production of testosterone by the Leydig cells in the testes is also controlled," he said.

"Although dietary control is always more difficult than simply taking a drug, it also has *no* negative side effects. In fact, controlling arachidonic acid will have some additional benefits, particularly at the level of another hormonal system known as eicosanoids, which are superhormones of the body that virtually control all of our physiological systems. Among other things, they control high blood pressure and the synthesis of structural proteins such as keratin, the major structural component of hair."

How do you keep this delicate balance? Dr. Sears explained that if you can achieve the right ratio of protein to carbohydrates in your diet, you will be able to control the eicosanoid hormones with druglike precision. In essence, he said, you will be treating food as if it were a prescription drug, delivering a controlled amount of protein and carbohydrates at every meal.

In my experience, and the experience of many other men, this has been effective in helping to control hair loss, especially in combination with herbs that inhibit the body's production of the hair-follicle-killing DHT and the drug finasteride (as Proscar or Propecia), which also inhibits DHT production.

Another plus when you modify your diet: When you eat foods that provide nutrients essential for the hair and scalp, and foods that will maximize the intake and absorption of these essential nutrients, you are also fighting hair loss and encouraging growth. A sugar-balancing diet does this too.

If you do not have male pattern baldness, food may not adversely affect your normal hair growth, but food *does* play a profound role in the lives of those who have inherited the gene that causes male pattern baldness.

What and How Should I Eat?

Staying clear of the average American diet is one of the best defenses against hair loss. A balance of lean protein sources, such as turkey, chicken, fish, red meat (only occasionally), and soy products; and complex carbohydrates from fruits, vegetables, and beans; plus monounsaturated fats from olive oil and certain nut oils (see the list below) will ensure that you'll have an effective dietary balance that can help with hair loss. By following the proper diet, you can vastly increase your chances of success when using drug or herbal therapies for hair loss.

CARBOHYDRATES

Do eat plenty of fruits, vegetables, and beans.

Don't eat potatoes, pasta, and bread on a regular basis. They immediately turn to glucose and dramatically throw insulin levels out of whack when your blood sugar rises very quickly, then falls. This threatens proper hormonal function. Keep these foods to a minimum in your diet.

MONOUNSATURATED FATS

Use only these oils, in their whole form as fruits/nuts, or as extracted oils: extra virgin olive, almond, avocado, macadamia, cashew, pistachio, pecan, and hazelnut.

ALCOHOL

Alcohol should only be used in moderation, and more than one drink per day is not advised. Heavy alcohol consumption robs the body of vital nutrients, including zinc, folic acid, vitamin C, and vitamin B. Alcohol acts as a diuretic and can cause severe dehydration, which directly affects the condition of the scalp, as well as hair growth. Alcohol also plays havoc with your blood-sugar levels and your hormones.

CAFFEINE

Limit your intake of caffeine. Long-term use of caffeine robs the body of vitamins B and C and the minerals potassium and zinc. This stresses the adrenal glands, which causes the depletion of vital nutrients in the bloodstream, which then adversely affects DHT levels.

NICOTINE

Avoid the use of nicotine. It depletes the body of important nutrients, and long-term use puts extreme stress on the adrenal glands.

KEEP YOUR BLOOD SUGAR BALANCED

- If you are not overweight, your body will make better use of its insulin.
- Eat five or six small meals a day: breakfast, lunch, and dinner, with a light snack between each meal and a nightly snack if desired or needed.
- Don't let more than three hours go by without eating something.
- Avoid refined and processed foods. Whole and natural foods are used by the body more slowly and evenly, which allows for steady blood-sugar levels.
- Avoid snacks and desserts that contain refined sugar, such as cakes, cookies, pastries, ice cream, candy, canned fruits, and the like.
- Soluble fiber, the kind found in vegetables, oats, and fruits, helps your intestines absorb glucose (sugar) in a steady, even manner.

- Reducing your salt intake reduces blood-sugar levels.
- Exercise lowers blood-sugar levels.
- Stress can cause fluctuations in blood-sugar levels.
- When your blood-sugar level is extremely low and you feel dizzy, light-headed, disoriented, or nauseated, drink eight ounces of orange juice. It will raise your blood-sugar level almost immediately and will also relieve symptoms in a few minutes.

To achieve the sugar-balancing effect in your diet, Dr. Sears recommends that in each meal you eat 30 percent protein, 40 percent complex carbohydrates, and 30 percent monounsaturated fats. You can further refine your diet by following the formulas in *The Zone,* which show you how to calculate your own unique protein requirements based on your weight, lean body mass, and activity level.

Using the 30-40-30 guideline, you can begin balancing your diet today and create a beneficial internal environment supportive of hair-loss prevention and regrowth, as well as an overall health-supporting way of eating.

3

THE POWER OF HERBAL TREATMENTS

We never stop investigating. We are
never satisfied that we know enough to
get by. Every question we answer leads
to another question. This has become
the greatest survival trick of our
species.

—DESMOND MORRIS

Scientific studies and clinical experience show
that a number of herbs, botanicals, and nutrients
can inhibit DHT, the testosterone derivative that
shrinks and ultimately kills hair follicles in people
with the gene for male pattern baldness.

In fact, some herbs inhibit the effects of DHT
as effectively as—and in many men even better
than—synthetic pharmaceutical drugs.

At least 20,000 scientific papers have been published in journals that attest to the efficacy of herbal, botanical, and nutritional intervention to both prevent and treat all manner of human ills.

"More than 25 percent of our mainstream pharmaceuticals are derived from plants, and 60 percent have additional plant-based ingredients," reports journalist and author Nina L. Diamond in her book *Purify Your Body: Natural Remedies for Detoxing from 50 Everyday Situations.* "We already know the chemical properties of many other herbs and botanicals that heal or positively affect the body and mind. These are used in natural treatments but aren't yet being synthesized into pharmaceuticals."

If herbs and botanicals work so well, why do drug companies bother to create synthetic versions of them, adding other chemicals in the process, and turn them into over-the-counter or prescription drugs?

The answer is very simple: You can't claim ownership of a plant, botanical, or nutrient and then patent it. For economic reasons, drug companies synthesize many of these natural substances and create a brand-new man-made compound, which they can then claim exclusive ownership of. The drug company obtains a patent for their new compound and is granted the right to be the only company that can sell the drug for a number of years, until the patent expires. After that, other drug companies can also manufacture and market the drug.

Faced with the growing competition from herbs, botanicals, and nutrients in their natural form, as their medicinal and healing properties are scientifically documented and more people are incorporating them into their health care, many pharmaceutical companies now have divisions that sell natural, herbal products. None of these can be exclusively owned by any one company, of course, so numerous brands are available, not only from divisions of pharmaceutical companies but from companies that do not manufacture and market pharmaceutical drugs, only herbal, botanical, and other natural products such as vitamins, minerals, and nutritional supplements.

"At least 20,000 scientific papers have been published in journals that attest to the efficacy" of herbal, botanical and nutritional intervention regarding health, Diamond notes. "In Europe, particularly Germany, scientists, medical researchers, physicians, and health practitioners are way, way ahead of the United States in this area."

The U.S. is working on catching up, however, and some of the research and clinical studies of natural treatments, including herbs, is now funded by the National Institutes of Health (NIH) through their Office of Alternative Medicine, which was created in 1992.

"Although the alternative forms of medicine are each unique, they are characteristically respectful of the body's inner self-correcting mechanisms, seeking to assist the body's natural and spontaneous healing intelligence," writes natural health activist and author John Robbins in his book *Reclaiming Our Health.*

What we call alternative medicine is actually our *original* medicine. Natural treatments have been the mainstay of medicine since time began. Before the advent of modern pharmaceuticals, barely one hundred years ago, they were the *only* medicine we had. Certainly, many of these synthesized pharmaceutical drugs are essential and life-saving, but natural treatments are just as vital to our health and well-being, and although herbs, botanicals, and nutrients are powerful (that's why they work) and should be used as carefully as drugs, these natural treatments often have the advantage of producing fewer side effects than synthetic drugs.

For the prevention and treatment of male pattern baldness, herbs, botanicals, and nutrients have been proven quite effective, and they can be used alone or in conjunction with other approaches such as pharmaceutical drugs and hair transplantation surgery.

Consult with a physician who is knowledgeable about natural medicine, such as a naturopathic physician, herbalist, or nutritionist, when choosing your preventive and treatment approaches.

When I became involved in helping others deal with their hair loss, I provided them with my experiences and information about the drug finasteride, which, when I started, was only available as Proscar, marketed as a DHT-reducing 5 mg. pill for prostate enlargement. Now, of course, it's available as Propecia, the DHT-reducing 1 mg. pill for the prevention and treatment of male pattern baldness.

Many people were asking me about effective natural, herbal methods that might also lower DHT levels or prevent DHT from affecting hair follicles. A number of natural, effective methods are available. I provided this information to them, adding that I was using herbs in conjunction with finasteride, and I had slowed my hair loss, experienced a lot of hair regrowth, and had no side effects.

Some of the men used the recommended herbs (saw palmetto, *Pygeum africanum,* and stinging nettle, or just saw palmetto alone) in conjunction with finasteride, while others used the herbal treatment alone. All experienced marked improvement.

"I thought that I may have been too quick to judge the herb treatment a success, but my hair still keeps growing," wrote Gary, who, at twenty-five years old, had already lost a significant amount of hair. "I am still totally amazed at this. I have tried various methods and began them all with the proper self-confidence and attitude you need, but ultimately they failed to deliver. To be honest, I did not put much faith in the idea of herbs. But they worked! I'm sorry if I sound excited, but that is because I am."

Jim, a Michigan man in his fifties, wrote: "I began taking *Pygeum* and saw palmetto. After only two months, my haircutter noticed new hair growth in the area on top that was thinning. After four to five months, the thinning area is approximately 50 percent filled in. I'm impressed with these results thus far and will continue with the herbal approach."

After seven months on saw palmetto, *Pygeum,* and nettle, Mario wrote: "I have been very happy with the results. I have had a dramatic decrease in hair fall-out and a much denser growth of hair. A small bald spot in the back of my head was completely filled in. I will continue this treatment indefinitely."

At thirty-two, Giovanni, of Carlos Casares, Argentina, had been experiencing gradual hair loss for seven years on the top of his head and at his front hairline.

"The excruciating torture of watching my hair

and my youth slowly vanish has been a painful experience," he wrote. "I am a basically skeptical person and do not pay much attention to money-grubbing sales pitches and scammers. The hair-loss prevention field is filled with such charlatans. That I was able to find you amidst this disreputable lot was nothing short of a miracle. Here at last was someone who gave me an honest appraisal of the available options, and who gave the understanding and support of someone who had experienced the anxieties and hurt involved in hair loss, and the disappointment and discouragement that comes with seeking help in a cruel world of rip-off artists. Through the information you provided me, I was able to make a decision to treat my hair loss through the natural herbs. Happily, this has resulted in considerable reduction in the amount of hair I am losing. I am also planning to start taking finasteride. Thanks to you, the only person who ever gave me honest advice in this business, I now know what my further options are and what the risks involved are."

Saw Palmetto (Serenosa repens)

Extract of the berries of the saw palmetto shrub protects the prostate, slows hair loss, and encourages hair regrowth by reducing the uptake of DHT by the hair follicles.

Unlike the drug finasteride, and the action of herbs that behave like finasteride, saw palmetto doesn't inhibit the enzyme 5-alpha-reductase, which converts testosterone to DHT. Saw palmetto, instead, prevents the hair-follicle-killing DHT from binding to the receptor sites at the prostate and the hair follicles.

"Saw palmetto has been used for centuries, first by Native Americans and later by European herbalists and naturopathic doctors. A considerable amount of research has documented its efficacy even when compared to the leading drug finasteride," reports naturopathic physician Joseph Pizzorno, N.D., founding president of Bastyr University, the first fully accredited multidisciplinary university of natural medicine in the United States and the site of research and studies into natural medicine funded by the National Institutes of Health, in his book *Total Wellness.* "Saw palmetto is effective in nearly 90 percent of patients, usually in four to six weeks, and has no negative side effects."

In *Purify Your Body,* Nina L. Diamond reports that "although mainstream physicians are slowly catching on to the value of saw palmetto, their patients and men in general are way ahead of them. The demand for the herb has increased so dramatically in recent years that farmers, pickers, and packers report a tremendous increase in production to keep up. Saw palmetto is native to the southeastern United States. Prices are reasonable, around $14.98 for a bottle of one hundred capsules, which, when you take two capsules a day as a preventive or for treatment, will provide you with almost a two-month supply."

Success with saw palmetto has prompted even more study.

"Saw palmetto research and study in the U.S. and Europe is one of the fastest-growing research areas, with excellent results," Diamond writes. "Many enlightened mainstream physicians have already incorporated saw palmetto into their prevention and treatment plans for their patients."

Not only does saw palmetto have no adverse side effects, but it has been used to treat impotence and increase virility. In a very small percentage of men, however, it can have the same libido-lowering effect as Propecia.

USING SAW PALMETTO

- Do *not* use the dried berries themselves, as they will not affect your DHT activity. Use only saw palmetto capsules (pills) made from the berry extract.
- The label *must* state the following informa-

tion: concentrated and purified; and 85–95 percent fatty acids and sterols (don't worry, these are *not* steroids). *Only extracts made to these specifications will work.*

- Take one 160 mg. pill twice each day. You can take one in the morning and one at night.
- Saw palmetto is nontoxic, has no known adverse side effects, and you can stay on it indefinitely.
- The extract will protect your prostate, helping to prevent inflammation, enlargement, infection, and cancer. It is also used to treat all of these conditions, so while you are taking saw palmetto to prevent and treat hair loss, you are also doing a good deed for your prostate.

Green Tea (Camellia sinensis)

Green tea contains catechins, a group of compounds that inhibit the enzyme Type I 5-alpha-reductase (which is predominantly in skin, while Type II is found in skin and the prostate), which converts testosterone into DHT.

In a chemical reaction like finasteride, then, green tea prevents the body's manufacture of

DHT. Finasteride does it through the Type II 5-alpha-reductase, however.

Because of its ability to keep your body from making its usual amount of DHT, green tea has been shown in published studies and clinical experience to be effective in preventing and treating male pattern baldness. Green tea is also rich in antioxidants, and the tea's active catechin compounds also lower cholesterol, have antibacterial action, and protect the cardiovascular system.

USING GREEN TEA

You can drink the tea, a delicious brew that is considered the national beverage of Japan, or take green tea in powdered form in capsules. Do not mistake this for the "regular" tea you may be used to drinking. Green tea is different, and it will be labeled specifically as green tea. It is made from the *unfermented* leaves of the tea plant. (The black tea you may be commonly drinking is the fermented version.) Green tea is nontoxic and has no adverse side effects.

Pygeum (Pygeum africanum)

Pygeum, an herb derived from the bark of the African evergreen, also inhibits the enzyme 5-alpha-reductase, which converts testosterone into hair-follicle-killing DHT, and is widely used in Europe to prevent and treat prostate problems and to prevent and treat male pattern baldness. Studies have shown that pygeum also improves male sexual function.

USING PYGEUM

- Take between 60 and 500 mg. per day in pill or capsule form.
- The label must say that the pygeum's beta sterol count is 13 percent. (Again, don't worry, the substance is sterol, *not* steroid!) The pygeum will not be effective if the count is less than 13 percent.
- Taking pygeum dosages along with your daily saw palmetto and stinging nettle dosages is a very effective combination.
- Stinging nettle (see below) enhances the pygeum's function and can be taken with it for maximum effect.

Stinging Nettle (Urtica dioica)

The Romans used the stinging nettle plant to improve virility, and in tea form it has long been used to help improve the health of your skin and hair.

USING STINGING NETTLE

- Stinging nettle enhances the effects of pygeum and can be taken in pill or capsule form.
- Take 50 to 100 mg. per day.

Zinc

Studies and clinical experience show that the mineral zinc inhibits the activity of 5-alpha-reductase and also inhibits the ability of testosterone and hair-follicle-killing DHT to bind to your cells' receptors, thereby protecting the follicles from DHT while also allowing for increased excretion of these hormones. It has been used successfully in prostate treatment and, because of its effects on 5-alpha-reductase, it also helps prevent and treat male pattern baldness.

USING ZINC

- Discuss with your doctor the dosages and length of time you'll be using zinc. For effective action against 5-alpha-reductase and DHT, zinc is used for six months at 60 mg. per day. For long-term use, your doctor can modify the dosage and give you a schedule.

- Use only Zinc Picolinate, which is the best-absorbed form of zinc.
- Zinc is taken in pill or capsule form.
- Many people have a zinc deficiency, which is even more common as we age, primarily because the body isn't able to absorb enough of the zinc it gets from food or from forms of zinc supplements other than Zinc Picolinate.

Essential Fatty Acids

Studies and clinical experience show that essential fatty acids (EFAs), including those found in linseed oil, sunflower oil, black currant oil (rich in GLA: gamma linolenic acid), evening primrose oil and soy oil, are effective against the processes that harm the prostate and contribute to male pattern baldness.

Essential fatty acids include linoleic, linolenic, and arachidonic acids (see Chapter Two for more on the role that arachidonic acids play in the body and hair loss). Oils that contain one or more of these are found frequently in our diet.

USING EFAS

One teaspoon per day of one of the above oils is all you'll need. While you can take black currant oil or evening primrose oil capsules, you can also use one teaspoon of sunflower oil with other dressing ingredients on a salad or other food and obtain the recommended dosage that way.

It's often hard to get enough GLA in your diet, and since it promotes healthy skin, hair, and nails and acts as an effective anti-inflammatory with none of the side effects of a prescription anti-inflammatory, it's an important substance. With just one 500 mg. capsule of black currant oil twice a day, you will notice an improvement in the texture, density, and quality of your hair in six to eight weeks.

Ho Shou Wu

A very well-known Chinese herb whose name translates to "Mr. Ho has black hair," Ho Shou Wu has long been used as a rejuvenating herb for the hair, as well as for overall energy, blood purifying, and to nourish the teeth and skin.

The herb can be found in Chinese herbal shops and natural health stores in both tea and capsule form.

4

A LOOK AT SURGICAL
SOLUTIONS

First, do no harm.
—FROM THE HIPPOCRATIC OATH

Most people considering hair transplantation are
not aware of the scope and the pitfalls of this medical specialty. While some patients may understand the basic science behind the procedure, few
have any grasp of the aesthetics and artistry required of the most demanding of all cosmetic procedures. Unfortunately, many of the physicians
who perform these procedures are as ill informed
as their patients.

Flashy marketing and high-pressure sales
pitches dominate the industry, making truly objective and rational decision-making by the patient

nearly impossible. Hair transplantation is handled not so much as the *medical specialty* that it is, one that serves *patients,* but as a *business* that serves *consumers.*

The aim of many of the physicians in the field is to confuse the prospective patient, which isn't very difficult since the patient is in such a desperate state about their hair loss to begin with. Although there are almost 200,000 physicians performing all sorts of so-called hair-restoration procedures in the United States, literally only a handful perform these procedures well and to safe, nondisfiguring, state-of-the-art specifications.

"The history of this industry has been less than forthcoming and open in its representations of the results obtained from the various hair-restoration procedures over the last thirty-plus years," says Dr. William R. Rassman, who, in 1995, in the *International Journal of Aesthetic and Restorative Surgery,* with his colleague Dr. Robert M. Bernstein, introduced follicular transplantation, the state-of-the-art technique now considered the safest, most natural-looking and successful hair-transplantation method. Rassman and Bernstein, through their breakthrough technique, published reports in medical journals, and presentations at medical conferences, have emerged as the field's visionaries and conscience. "Much of the lack of openness still exists. For this reason, you should be wary of dubious medical claims and results that do not allow direct examination by meeting and examining patients directly. The more primitive techniques of the past will hopefully be laid to rest sooner rather than later."

As a consumer advocate, I speak with people in various stages of the hair-loss process, including those who have already undergone hair-restoration surgery. Most of these people are unhappy with the results, and many even feel that they have been deformed (and indeed many of them *have*) by outdated surgical procedures still being performed by lazy, unscrupulous physicians. I have personally seen horrific deformities caused by such barbaric procedures as flaps, scalp reductions, linear grafts, and hair lifts.

Many physicians are still using outdated methods of hair transplantation, leaving the patient with a pluggy, unnatural look (resembling doll hair) and a great deal of scalp-deforming scarring called *cobblestoning* that occurs around the implants.

Do *not* agree to any of the following seven outdated procedures.

1. *Flap*

A flap of skin with its tissue, hair strands, and hair follicles is shifted from the side of the head to the front hairline by cutting it on three sides, thus not separating it from its blood supply or severing it completely from the scalp. The procedure is major surgery and is performed in a hospital. A flap is one inch wide and approximately three to seven inches long. It has to be twisted in order for the hair side of the flap to end up facing outward from the head once it's been flopped over and stitched to the balding area. A knot will form at this twist and leave a lumpy look. Other serious problems with this procedure include:

- Necrosis: a very high chance of partial or complete death of the flap, leaving a wide, ugly scar.
- Hair grows in the opposite direction than normal.
- Infection.
- Hair loss and extreme scarring in the donor area.
- Loosened skin in the forehead develops and hangs over the brow, giving a Frankenstein or Neanderthal appearance.
- Absence of hair behind the newly created frontal hairline.
- Poor positioning of the flap.
- Scarring at stitching of the flap.
- Integrity of the scalp is compromised.

A type of flap known as the free-form flap is created when all four sides are cut and the flap is completely removed from the donor area so that in its new position in the balding area it can be set in the direction of natural growth. Neither the flap nor the free-form flap procedure should ever be done.

2. Linear or Line Grafts

A 3–4 mm linear strip of donor hair is removed from the side or back of the head, and instead of dividing the strip into tiny grafts the entire strip or large parts of it are transplanted. Since this large graft can't be placed into tiny holes, a trench is surgically cut into the bald area and the graft is placed in the trench. As the hair grows, it looks like a line of hair and is not cosmetically acceptable.

3. Round or Square Grafts

These are the original, standard, out-of-date, pluggy-looking grafts. Each 3–5 mm graft is made with a hole-punch device, resulting in a plug of

75

hair about the size of a pencil eraser. Whether these large grafts are round or square, they are too large and do not even remotely resemble the way hair naturally grows from the head. When transplanted, because the grafts are so large and therefore compromise the blood supply, hair in the middle of the graft often does not grow, leaving the patient with a doughnut effect. These large grafts are responsible for what looks like doll hair—a pluggy look of islands of hair in an ocean of baldness, as they are now described. Cobblestoning is very common with this procedure. Even the more recently developed smaller versions of these grafts—the mini grafts and the micro grafts—can give a less than natural appearance, which is why it is recommended that transplants should be comprised of only tiny grafts called *follicular units*, clusters of the one-to-four hairs that grow naturally this way in your scalp. (See entire section on the follicular transplantation procedure, pages 87 to 89.)

4. Scalp Reduction

Also known as alopecia reduction (AR), galeoplasty (GP), or male pattern reduction (MPR), scalp reductions are barbaric and disfiguring. Performed in the doctor's office under local anesthesia, the bald part of the scalp at the top or crown of the head is literally cut away, and the edges of the nearby hairy skin are sewn together, bringing the hair-bearing scalp from either side to meet in the middle. In some cases, a hideous scar results that makes the top or back of your head look like your buttocks. The scalp reduction scar is sitting in the middle of an area in which scalp is still often seen, resembling the "crack" between the two cheeks you sit on. Scalp reduction problems also include:

- Accelerated hair loss, more than the natural course your hair loss would take. This hair loss can occur within only weeks or months, and that hair often doesn't return.
- Thinning of the scalp.
- An unnatural appearance because direction of hair growth is altered.
- Infection.
- Hemorrhaging and hematoma (blood pooling).
- Stretch back, in which the stretched part of the hair-bearing scalp that has been stitched together loses its tightness and stretches out partially or totally, leaving a visible scar-tissue bald area created by the stretching, revealing the buttocks "crack" scar.

- Suture reaction, in which the stitches in the deep layers below the skin can cause pain and swelling. The body can reject the sutures, causing holes in the scalp at the suture sites.

- Scalp reductions do not preserve hair for use in transplants, as some physicians may try to claim, for the same wreath of permanent hair is stretched to cover a wider area in the crown, thereby thinning the permanent hair that would normally be used as donor hair for transplantation.

5. Hair Lift

This is a more radical form of the scalp reduction, in which dissection or loosening of the scalp skin is done at a level below the major arteries of the scalp. To avoid damaging these blood vessels, the nerves are cut and tied. *This leaves your head permanently numb.* Unlike other scalp reductions, this is major surgery, which requires hospitalization and general anesthesia. It leaves visible scars around the ears, and additional hair loss is often a consequence of this ill-advised procedure.

6. *Scalp Expanders*

These are silicone balloons that are inserted into pockets that are created between the inside of your scalp and your skull. After the incisions heal, in several weeks, the balloons are gradually inflated with a series of salt-solution injections. The head is blown up to two or three times its normal size. This radical procedure is only recommended in trauma cases when the patient has received deep burns to the scalp.

All other forms of scalp expansion, except for use in trauma cases, is not recommended.

7. *The Use of a Dilator*

After creating the tiny slit that the transplanted hair will fit into, some doctors insert a *dilator*, a hollow steel pin that resembles a straw. They remove the dilator and then place the tiny hair graft into the dilator-widened slit. The disadvantages include the following:

- Many doctors are unable to control the direction in which the transplanted hair will grow when dilators are used.

- The recipient-site tissue can be damaged by the dilator.
- Recipient-site pinholes have to be more widely spaced to accommodate the width of the dilators. This results in less dense hair coverage.

"As grafts became smaller, some doctors had great difficulty placing the delicate grafts into the small holes or micro slits in the recipient area of the scalp," explains Dr. William Rassman. "Some doctors started using dilators. These steel pins are placed, often with some pressure, so that the doctors or technicians could locate the holes for graft placement. With time, however, many doctors have learned that these dilators were not necessary and that the grafts could be placed into the holes without them. What was required was a learning curve, something that some doctors choose *not* to learn."

Regarding this issue, Dr. Rassman cautions against physicians who are less skilled at the delicate transplantation procedure. "If doctors can't do the procedure with a delicate touch, then telling the patient that dilators are the only way to do hair transplantation is like an artist telling his clients that only house brushes can paint a fine Mona Lisa," he quips.

* * *

"It seems that anyone who declares themselves hair-transplant specialists seems to be able to promote themselves to a vulnerable and naive public, even with little experience or training in the area," Dr. Rassman cautioned in the July 1994 issue of *Hair Transplant Forum International,* the official publication of the International Society of Hair Restoration Surgery. "Moving from the standard hair-transplant quantities with larger grafts to very large quantities of very *small* grafts is a significantly more complex and intricate process than most practitioners realize."

The aim of this chapter is to safely walk the patient through this treacherous minefield of an industry. Keep in mind that many of these unscrupulous physicians, their medical assistants, and salespeople will say or do anything to "make the sale."

The information on surgical techniques provided in this chapter is the most up-to-date and state-of-the-art and will give a most natural appearance with no deformities, scarring, pluggy look, or cobblestoning. This chapter highlights the work of those two physicians who are considered the voice and conscience of this completely unregulated industry. I have researched Dr. Bernstein's and Dr. Rassman's groundbreaking follicular-transplant techniques and interviewed countless physicians, and as Dr. O'Tar

Norwood (famed for the Norwood Scale, which decades ago set the standard for measuring male pattern baldness) writes in the May 1997 issue of *Hair Transplant Forum International,* Bernstein's and Rassman's methodology is "an idea whose time has come."

With careful research, and the information provided in this book about advances in techniques, hair transplantation should be completely undetectable and natural looking. I strongly urge anyone who is considering hair-transplantation surgery to consider physicians recommended in the Resource Guide at the end of the book, and those physicians they can recommend in your area.

When hair transplantation is used alone or as an adjunct to drugs, diet, or herbal therapies, it may very well be possible to safely retain or restore a healthy, attractive head of hair for life.

Hair-Transplant Basics

Before walking you through the hair-transplant procedure or discussing the follicular-transplantation method in depth, let's take a look at some of the basics regarding hair transplantation:

- Hair transplants can only be performed by donating your *own* hair to your head from your *own* donor areas, or between identical twins. Otherwise your body will reject the transplanted hair, follicle, and tissue.
- The hair on the sides and back of the head remains even in those with extensive male pattern baldness, who will just end up with thinner sides and back. These areas are the *donor sites* from which *donor hair* is extracted and transplanted to other parts of the scalp into tiny slits created by the doctor's surgical tools.
- The donated hair, hair follicles, surrounding tissue, and skin are called *grafts*.
- Each graft contains one or more hair follicles, with accompanying hair, tissue, and skin.
- No two heads are alike.
- The *art* of hair transplantation is as important as the medical technique.
- *Hair density* is the number of hair follicles per square centimeter of scalp.
- *Scalp laxity* is the flexibility and looseness of the scalp. The more flexible your scalp, the better.
- More hair can be transplanted when the scalp is loose and the density is high.
- Hair grows in different directions on differ-

ent parts of the head: forward at the *front and top,* down or away from the *middle of the head on the sides,* and back and down in the *rear.*

- *Coarse hair* has greater bulk and can be transplanted with fewer hairs per graft. Coarse hair also gives greater coverage.
- *Fine hair* has less bulk and gives very natural but less coverage than coarse hair.
- *Curly and wavy hair* gives good results more easily in hair transplantation because a single curly hair curls on itself and covers more scalp than a straight hair. Curly hair also holds its shape and rises from the scalp, again giving the appearance of greater coverage.
- *Straight hair* lies against the scalp and gives a less dense appearance in coverage than curly or wavy hair.
- The closer the *hair color* is to the *skin color,* the better the appearance of coverage. African hair is dark, very curly, and provides the least contrast against various shades of dark skin. This produces the best transplant results visually. Fair-haired men with a fair complexion also have a low contrast between hair and skin shades. This produces excellent results. Asian men with dark, straight hair and a beige complexion have a

higher contrast between hair and skin shades and pose the most artistic challenges in hair transplantation. Excellent results can be achieved, though, by a highly skilled surgeon.

- When designing the procedure, the doctor must consider the patient's future hair-loss pattern and rate of change.
- Design of the hairline and choosing the recipient sites for the transplanted hair are important considerations. Transplants are artistically planned, and natural hairlines vary from person to person.
- By using tiny *follicular units* (one to four hairs in naturally occurring clusters), doctors can begin transplanting hair in the early stages of hair loss and when hair is first receding.
- The front and top of the head receive transplanted hair first. The crown is saved for last unless it's the patient's only balding area.
- You can often get desired results in one or two transplant sessions if they are long sessions, in which thousands of hairs are transplanted in follicular units of one to four hairs each. Future transplant sessions can follow the progression of hair loss if necessary.
- Each hair-transplant session can last between five and ten hours.

THE PRELIMINARY EXAM

During your first consultation with the doctor who will perform your hair-transplant procedure, he should do the following:

- Give you a thorough physical examination of your head and take a detailed pertinent medical history.
- The examination of your head should include the use of a Hair Densitometer™, an instrument that measures your hair density and allows the doctor to evaluate the number of hairs in each of your naturally occurring follicular units and the eventual hair-loss pattern you might experience over time. Your fine hairs are also compared to your thick ones. This measures the degree of miniaturization of your hair strands caused by shrinking hair follicles, which is the progressive diminishing of the hair's diameter and length.
- The doctor should put in writing your transplant design and estimated timetable for your procedures.
- The doctor should clearly explain the entire transplant procedure and any and all associated risks.

Keep in mind that when you go in for your consultation you have to have something to show the doctor, and that means don't go in with a shaved head or a buzz cut. Let the hair grow out a bit before having your consultation.

The Follicular Transplantation Procedure

Hair transplantation surgery takes many hours and involves not only the doctor but a number of medical technicians and nurses. Performed in the doctor's office, these procedures require only a local anesthesia: a mild sedative followed by injections in the scalp to numb the donor and recipient areas, similar to the novocaine shots you receive during a dental procedure.

The patient can either be reclining or lying down during the procedure, and often listening to music or chatting with the medical staff.

Let's take a step-by-step look at what happens after the patient has received the local anesthesia.

1. A strip of donor scalp is chosen by the doctor. Hair on the strip is cut short, and then, using a scalpel, the doctor removes the strip of scalp from the donor area on the side or back of the head. The donor strip is placed in a container filled with a chilled saline solution or Ringer's lactate.

2. The donor area is stitched closed. Do *not* use a doctor who leaves the donor site open. An

open wound, no matter how large or small, will greatly increase the chances of scarring. Hair above the donor site will help cover the stitched donor area. The site will heal within a week or two, and afterward the stitches will be removed unless the doctor has used dissolvable stitches. The process leaves a fine scar that is virtually undetectable under the surrounding hair.

3. The strip of donor scalp is dissected under a microscope and trimmed of extra fatty tissue by the medical technicians. This is a long, detailed, and exacting process, so while parts of the donor strip are being dissected and then implanted, other parts lie in wait in a refrigerator set at 40° F. During the dissection process, the donor scalp is cut into *follicular units* of one to four hairs each. These are naturally occurring individual hair groups. Each unit (whether it's a one-hair, two-hair, three-hair, or four-hair unit) includes the hair strand(s), the hair follicle(s), and some of the surrounding tissue and skin. Great care must be taken not to damage the follicles.

4. The overall recipient site—the area of your scalp that will receive the transplants—has already been chosen during a presurgery examination with your doctor. During the surgical procedure, the doctor will draw on your scalp the outline of the area receiving the transplants. This outline may be your soon-to-be created frontal hairline, the area at the top or crown. Each individual recipient site

is prepared to receive the transplant graft when a very tiny slit is created with a small, specialized scalpel.

5. The hair grafts of follicular units are then placed into the recipient sites in the proper direction of natural hair growth.

After the first session, future transplant surgeries should involve removal of the original scar from the previous session's donor site and the harvesting of an adjacent section from the donor site in order to minimize the number of scarred locations under the hair. Otherwise a series of scars could cause a stepladder appearance in the donor areas if the hair covering the scars is very thin.

Doctors should place the grafts into your scalp in the manner in which your hair would naturally grow so you can style it any way you choose and so that it will look natural even when it's not combed. Those who have low hair density or extensive balding and little donor hair may have transplants done in what's called a "weighted" manner, in which more hair is transplanted into one area than another to accommodate a hairstyle that gives good coverage. In any event, good hairstyling enhances all transplants.

FOLLICULAR TRANSPLANTATION

In 1984 pathologist John Headington described hair as growing in natural clusters of one to four hairs each and named these *follicular units.* During the late 1980s, Dr. Bobby L. Limmer, a San Antonio, Texas, physician, introduced the use of the microscope in hair-transplantation surgery. This very important contribution made the careful dissection of intact follicular units, as well as mini grafts and micro grafts, possible.

Robert M. Bernstein, M.D., assistant clinical professor of dermatology at the College of Physicians and Surgeons of Columbia University in New York and a practicing physician performing hair transplants, suggested that these naturally occurring follicular units should be used exclusively for the entire procedure. With his colleague William R. Rassman, M.D., a visionary, innovative Los Angeles surgeon and the inventor and holder of numerous patents in biotechnology (including the Hair Densitometer™, which measures hair density), a major breakthrough followed: The two decided that these units shouldn't be broken apart during transplantation but should, instead, be used in their naturally occurring one-, two-, three-, and four-hair groupings.

Hair-transplantation surgery took a giant leap forward in 1995 when Bernstein and Rassman refined the procedure. Bernstein named it follicular transplantation, and the two introduced it in the *International Journal of Aesthetic and Restorative Surgery* (vol. 3, no. 2).

"Follicular transplantation is the logical end

point of over thirty years of evolution in hair-restoration surgery, beginning with the traditional large plugs and culminating in the movement of one-, two-, and three-hair units, which mirror the way hair grows in nature," they wrote. "The key to follicular transplantation is to identify the patient's natural hair groupings, dissect the follicular units from the surrounding skin, and place these units in the recipient site in a density and distribution appropriate for a mature individual."

Prior to this, transplants were performed by moving groups of hair in large plugs of up to twenty hairs each into each recipient opening. The result was not cosmetically pleasing or natural looking. Hair simply does not naturally sprout from your head in large plugs.

Bernstein's and Rassman's new technique also solved many other problems associated with the older transplantation methods.

"The critical elements of follicular transplantation are an accurate estimation of the donor supply of hair, meticulous dissection of the follicular units, careful design of the recipient area to maximize the cosmetic impact of the transplant, the use of large numbers of implants in fewer rather than more sessions, a long-term master plan that accounts for the progression of the male pattern alopecia, and realistic expectations on the part of the patient," they reported.

Mirroring nature was the key.

"Hair emerges from the scalp in naturally occurring groups called *follicular units.* The surgeon can create hair patterns the way they grow in nature," says Dr. Rassman. Once transplanted, "these small grafts are often indistinguishable from the natural groups of hair growing in adjacent areas of the scalp."

Follicular units have between one and four hairs. These are the natural-growing groups of hair follicles and hair. The difference between older transplant procedures "and the state of the art today relates to the size and configuration" of the grafts, and from a visual point of view "this difference is as dramatic as day and night," Rassman says.

Previously, grafts were classified as *standard grafts, mini grafts,* and *micro grafts.* None mimic the way hair naturally grows from the head, and unfortunately, all three are still used by many doctors in transplantation procedures.

Standard grafts are those large plugs of hair that produce the most offensive doll-hair look. Ranging from 3 to 4 mm in diameter, with twelve to twenty or more hairs per graft, they are the look most associated with hair transplantation until recently.

Mini grafts were a slight improvement, ranging from 1.2 to 2.5 mm in diameter, with five to nine hairs per graft.

Micro grafts are a marked improvement but still inferior to today's state-of-the-art follicular units. Ranging in size from 1.0 to 1.5 mm in diameter, with only one to three hairs per graft, they were not created from natural arrangements of hair strands and their accompanying follicles—that is, not from naturally occurring follicular units. The natural-growing groups were instead ignored, "broken apart, and the subsequent damage to many follicles caused a high growth failure rate" after transplantation, says Dr. Rassman.

"Hair-restoration surgery is the single most common cosmetic surgical procedure performed in men in the U.S. and is still growing at a substantial rate," Bernstein and Rassman reported in the medical journal *Dermatologic Surgery* in 1997. "Of all cosmetic procedures in men, hair-restoration surgery has the potential to produce the most dramatic change in one's appearance. However, in no other form of cosmetic surgery has the road to achieving a desired result been more difficult for the patient. Problems produced by earlier surgical procedures which resulted in partial, incomplete, or distorted appearances over multiple-staged sessions often outweighed the long-term benefits."

It has been a long road to acceptable surgical results.

"The protracted course of traditional transplant surgeries that included 2 to 5 mm grafts, scalp reductions, or flaps, used alone or in combination, often produced significant disfigurement," they note. "By using follicular units exclusively in the transplants, the surgeon can safely move large quantities of implants in a single session and can create hair patterns that most closely mimic nature."

Like cosmetic or reconstructive surgery of any kind, hair transplantation should not leave the patient looking like a surgical road map but like the improvements were an original gift of nature.

"In the ideal situation, hair-restoration surgery should maintain the patient's adult appearance and give him the same 'look' as he would have had if he had simply 'matured,'" without extensive hair loss, they explain.

However, "the surgery should never attempt to restore the patient's adolescent appearance," they caution.

Commenting upon Bernstein's and Rassman's report in *Dermatologic Surgery*, Dr. Richard C. Shiell of Melbourne, Australia, applauded their advances. "There is no doubt that their techniques are revolutionizing hair-restoration surgery," he wrote, "and almost every practitioner in this field has already been influenced by their past writings and very convincing case presentations."

Despite such drastic improvements in techniques, many doctors continue to perform outdated, unacceptable procedures, and Dr. Rassman explains that this "issue is really one of change and the economics of this change. Change does not come easily to the established hair transplanters, but the results of traditional hair transplants have been so bad and so unnatural that the poor unfortunate patients who have received them have been unable to lead normal lives. The harm created from traditional transplantation techniques is the issue, and to argue it one must be blind. Perpetuating the present standard of care which produces substandard results defies logic and undermines our integrity as physicians."

Since hair transplantation has been seen as a good business opportunity in the eyes of some physicians who have neither the desire nor the skill to master the delicate technique, these opportunistic physicians are reluctant to embrace recent procedural advances.

"For those [doctors] who do not get good results, the focus should be on how to achieve them, or one should abandon performing the procedure altogether," says Dr. Rassman. "Our patients demonstrate a standard which we feel should become the standard of care. This is not a Rassman standard, it is nature's standard. Hair grows in units consisting of one to four hairs each and they should be transplanted that way."

An ideal hair transplant consists of follicular

units placed closely together. Hybrid grafting and blend grafting are different names for a two-technique process in which large grafts are used for the majority of the transplanted area, while the tiny, natural groups of follicular units are used only for the very visible front of the hairline. This technique is *not* recommended, as results are not as natural as using just follicular units.

ADVANTAGES TO FOLLICULAR TRANSPLANTS

In contrast to the larger, unnatural grafts, follicular units in transplant procedures provide the following medical and visual advantages:

- The surgical incision at each recipient site is smaller, therefore healing is quicker.
- Skin-surface deformity and scarring is eliminated because grafts and incisions are so small.
- A natural, not pluggy or doll-hair, appearance.
- Graft growth is superior.
- No cobblestoning scars at recipient site. These were commonly found in surgeries involving larger grafts and incisions.
- The size of each graft is based on the natural characteristics of the patient's hair since it is

determined by the naturally occurring follicular units.

- Natural scalp contour is preserved.
- Oxygen diffusion into implants is maximized.
- Interruption of normal blood flow to the grafts is minimized in the healing phase.
- Postoperative recovery time is greatly reduced.
- Hair units may be placed very close together because they are so small.
- Large numbers of implants may be moved per session.
- Hair may be distributed in a natural pattern.
- Great flexibility in designing recipient site areas.

LASERS IN HAIR TRANSPLANTATION

Some doctors have introduced the use of ultra- or super-pulsed CO_2 lasers into the transplantation procedure to create the holes at the recipient sites that the hair grafts will be inserted into. This has created some controversy because of the following considerations:

- Local anesthesia must be used at the recipient site, as in all hair-transplantation procedures, because the laser causes extreme pain.

When doctors advertise the laser as "painless," that claim is misleading. It is never used without first numbing the recipient site in the scalp.

- When laser sites are compared to sites made with scalpels, some patients have shown less hair growth in some of the laser-created sites. This is because the current lasers in use compromise proper oxygenation of the transplanted graft by reducing blood flow to the area.

- Heat damage in tissue surrounding the recipient sites becomes a concern as the number of grafts transplanted increases.

- Hair grafts may fall out of laser-created sites because the normal skin elasticity is affected by the laser's destruction of the skin collagen and elastic fibers.

- Laser-created sites produce more scarring and more tissue death.

- Healing progresses more slowly after laser transplantation.

- Regardless of how sophisticated or precise the laser becomes, it still destroys tissue and will therefore always be inferior to using a scalpel.

As Bernstein and Rassman note in the journal *Lasers in Surgery and Medicine* (vol. 19, no. 2,

1996), lasers are actually a new technology designed initially to work with an archaic technique—creating large, deep slits for the outdated and inferior-looking large hair plugs in procedures that are unfortunately still being performed by some doctors.

In follicular transplantation, however, large slits are *not* required in order "to accept the donor grafts. By identifying the patient's natural hair groupings, the implants can be pretrimmed of the excess tissue between the groups, resulting in tiny follicular units that can be placed in very small sites, solving the problems of both recipient bulkiness and compression," they explain. "Therefore, the claim that lasers have the advantage of removing recipient tissue while creating a slit has *no* relevance in follicular transplantation."

DESIGNING THE LOOK OF THE TRANSPLANTED SITE

Men with a substantial amount of hair left on their heads have a great deal of flexibility in terms of transplantation design.

A very bald man who doesn't have a high density of hair in the back or on the side donor areas has three options for transplant design: a thin layer of hair over all the bald areas, including desired hairline; a higher hairline, with moderate coverage in other previously bald areas; or the "forward weighting" method, in which donor hair creates the desired hairline framing the face and with moderate top coverage, but the crown is left bald or thin. This is the most aesthetically pleasing of the three options.

No matter how extensive your hair loss is, certain design considerations are essential in *every* transplant.

Bernstein and Rassman detail these and other transplant issues in the medical journal *Dermatologic Surgery* (vol. 23, no. 9, 1997), in a report that Dr. Shiell critiqued in that issue as "a most important work that should be essential reading for everyone performing hair-restoration surgery."

The transition zone is of prime importance when creating the new design of transplanted hair.

"The transition zone is the region that leads one's eye from the totally bald scalp into the thickness of the transplant. It is the most visible part of the reconstruction and therefore the most critical. As in other aspects of the transplant, the key to establishing a natural-looking transition zone is to mimic as closely as possible the one that occurs in nature," Bernstein and Rassman note. "Fortunately, follicular implants provide us with the tools to accomplish this."

Transition zones are visible in these locations:

the frontal hairline; the temples; the balding crown; and the sides, if the forelock becomes isolated.

Bernstein and Rassman explain that "a transition zone is also needed for the integration of transplanted hair into an area of existing hair and to camouflage larger grafts or plugs" that the patient may have from previous outdated transplants that resulted in the unacceptable, artificial, pluggy look.

"If one carefully observes a frontal hairline, one does not see a 'line' but a soft, feathery zone produced by a gradation of follicular units of increasing size and density," they report. "A natural-looking hairline can be created by the delicate placement of single hairs, followed by two-, three-, and possibly four-hair follicular units, depending upon the patient's density. This hair must always be harvested and implanted in the naturally occurring follicular groups for maximum growth and the best cosmetic result."

They caution, however, that the single-hair follicular units used at the front of the hairline should come from naturally occurring single-hair units, generally *not* from the dissection of larger units.

"Follicular units of two and three hairs should *not* be divided into single hairs, as this will increase the risk of poor growth," they note.

For the most natural appearance, doctors must remember that "another characteristic of the transition zone is that it is extremely irregular and often asymmetric. Since 'beauty' in all living things is defined, in part, by 'symmetry,' there must be a delicate balance between creating a zone that is 'too perfect' and one that does not maximally enhance the patient's appearance," they caution.

THE GROWTH OF TRANSPLANTED HAIR

The hair that has been placed in your recipient sites has been trimmed very short. It is quite common for "shock fall-out" to occur, in which these hairs and the original nontransplanted hairs (if any) within the recipient areas fall out soon after transplantation. This is only temporary, and your original hair as well as your newly transplanted hair *will return* in a normal growth cycle.

"The normal follicular growth cycle is quite variable," Bernstein and Rassman note in the medical journal *Dermatologic Surgery* (vol. 23, no. 9, 1997). "In most patients, the majority of the transplanted hair begins to grow at about three to four months after surgery, with additional hair appearing over the next several months. In a small percentage of patients, the onset of growth of the bulk of the hair can be seen from four to eight months or more, with additional new hair occasionally appearing up to eighteen months after the transplant."

Hair growth is not constant; it naturally occurs "within a few weeks, sometimes months, between growth spurts," they report. "Newly transplanted hair will increase in diameter and length."

If you are planning any other transplant sessions to follow your first one, wait at least eight to twelve months so that your previously transplanted hair has a chance to grow out.

As has been noted elsewhere in this chapter, some doctors are slow in adapting to the new, state-of-the-art procedures in hair-restoration surgery, and some are downright reluctant.

Michael D. Sparkhul, M.D., a Santa Paula, California, physician, has commented that adapting to the use of very tiny grafts takes enormous skill and commitment.

"These are long, tedious, extremely demanding procedures which, while they give some of the finest results I've ever seen, are not for the cavalier who expect to do an occasional case and get it right," he states simply. "It is *not* a procedure to be taken lightly. It requires herculean commitment, organization, and skill. The more I perform this procedure, the more it humbles me. One must be constantly vigilant."

The patient must be equally vigilant in his education about hair transplantation and in his choice of doctor.

5

HAIR SYSTEMS

In the middle of difficulty lies
opportunity.

     —ALBERT EINSTEIN (WHO HAD SOME
         HEAD OF HAIR)

We are so sensitive about hair loss that we have
come up with the politically correct term *hair system* to replace those good, old-fashioned words
hairpiece and *toupee,* so we can pretend that we're
using a *system,* instead of what we're really doing:
putting bought hair on our heads.

You'll remember those classic Hair Club for
Men television commercials: Not once was it ever
mentioned that this was about hairpieces or
weaves. It seemed to be a club that, when you
joined, hair would magically appear on your head.

Before I found the treatment that would slow my hair loss and cause regrowth, I considered that one day I might be in the market for a hairpiece, and that's when I began my research.

Hairpiece Foundation

The foundation for a hairpiece is made with either a section of netting that is cut and molded to fit the shape of the balding area you'll be covering, or silicone that is shaped to your head, or both.

Both the netting and silicone foundations can be attached with various forms of adhesive or clips, so you can remove the hairpiece as often as you want.

The silicone foundation is the most natural looking of the two foundations.

When netting is used as the foundation, hairs, individually or in tiny groups, are tied around the threads of the netting and knotted so they follow the hair's natural growth pattern.

The Hair in a Hairpiece

The best hairpieces are custom-made out of excellent-quality human hair matched to the hair of the client. This matching includes the color, texture, nature of curl or wave, or straightness, as well as hair density (thickness).

The hairs of less expensive hairpieces may either be made of a moderate-quality human hair, animal hair, or artificial fibers.

Most expensive and midpriced hairpieces are made from European hair that once grew naturally in a wide variety of colors, textures, densities, and levels of curl, wave, or straightness.

The least expensive hairpieces are made from dark, straight Asian hair that has been dyed or bleached. Although Asian hair is very strong, the coloring processes make it brittle and dry, so it breaks easily, and these hairpieces begin to look fuzzy very quickly and need to be replaced at frequent intervals.

Hairpieces are the most popular method of hair replacement, but the cost and appearance of any given hairpiece varies widely based on the materials used and the level of craftsmanship in their creation.

Human hair is fragile, so even the most expensive and expertly made hairpiece needs regular maintenance and needs to be replaced after a time.

Attaching the Hairpiece

Keep in mind that the way you attach your hairpiece will greatly affect the hair that may be directly under it or adjacent to it. A hairpiece can accelerate hair loss on the part of your head directly underneath it. Especially those hairpieces that are attached by bonding, a strong glue kind of adhesive, or are attached by the weaving process. Clips cause minimal hair loss.

PERMANENTLY ATTACHED HAIRPIECES

Hairpieces that are permanently attached are not designed to be removed except by a hair technician or stylist, usually once every six weeks. This can be very unhealthy for you, your head, and your hair. Shampooing can't remove the natural accumulation of flaked-off skin cells, oil, shed hair, and other organic debris that accumulates between the hairpiece and the scalp. Even if you have this kind of hairpiece, whether it's attached by bonding or weaving (in which your hair is woven into the bottom of the hairpiece in order to secure it to your head), it must be loosened or removed at least once every five days so you can properly clean the scalp underneath.

ADHESIVE-ATTACHED HAIRPIECES

Double-sided tape is used to attach the hairpiece. This is an easy kind of attachment, and you can remove it any time you want and then reattach it. It can, however, leave a sticky residue on your scalp and on the underside of the hairpiece, which you'll need to wash off. The tape can come unglued when you perspire heavily, and swimming loosens the tape as well.

CLIP ATTACHMENT

Metal clips that are securely attached to the underside of the hairpiece fasten to your own hair that's either under or adjacent to the hairpiece. These are secure but very easy to remove, just like tape attachment.

SNAP ATTACHMENT

Metal snaps are securely attached to the underside of the hairpiece, and these are then tied or sewn to your hair underneath or adjacent to the hairpiece. The snaps have to be relocated as your hair grows, and this kind of hairpiece attachment makes daily removal impossible. They are removed only by a technician. Like the permanent methods of attachment, using a snap attachment has a big downside regarding the health of your scalp and hair, since regular cleansing of the scalp isn't possible.

Weaves

Yes, weaves are what the Hair Club for Men is actually advertising.

During the weave process, strands of your own hair are pulled through the openings in the hairpiece's foundation and woven through it to secure the hairpiece to your head. There are many points of attachment, so a hair-weave attachment is very secure.

The hairpiece will need to be readjusted as your hair grows. Weaves often pull on your hair, and this can lead to further loss of the hair underneath the hairpiece. Weaves can cause *traction alopecia,* localized premature hair loss caused by pulling.

Again, weaves can be a problem regarding the health of the scalp, since the hairpiece is left in place for weeks at a time.

Tunnel Grafts

In this process, tunnels of skin are created in your scalp. These tunnels are made from your own skin with grafts surgically removed from another part of your body.

Three tunnels are created: one in front and two in back.

Your hairpiece will have plastic or nylon hooks sewn in, and these hooks will then be inserted into the tunnels on your head. Although this is a secure method of attachment, and the hairpieces are easy

The photographs in this section are representative of the types of results that can be achieved with the use of Propecia, Toppik, and Follicular Transplantation. Also included are some casualties of this unregulated industry. Unfortunately, this type of work has been the standard for years. Luckily, you don't have to be one of the casualties.

Propecia Successes

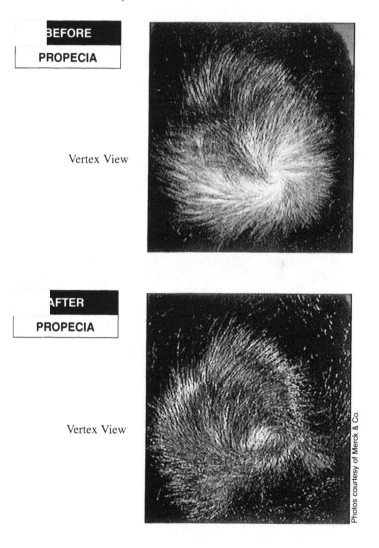

BEFORE

PROPECIA

Vertex View

AFTER

PROPECIA

Vertex View

Photos courtesy of Merck & Co.

Propecia Successes

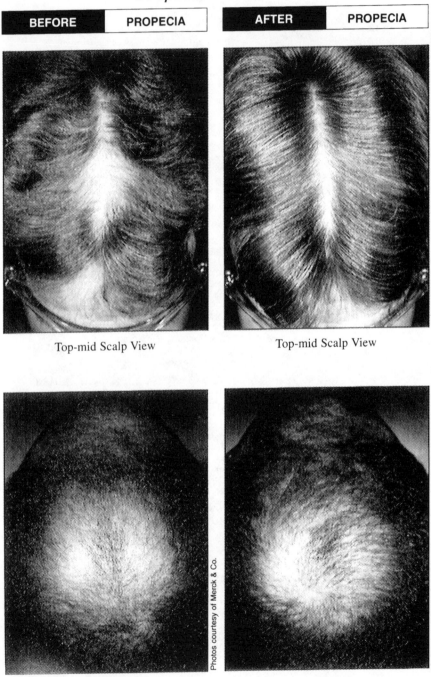

Hair Replacement Successes

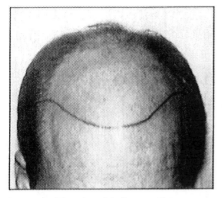

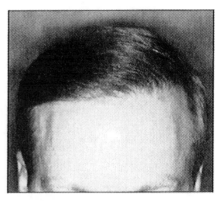

38-year-old male with front and top balding (Norwood Class 5a/6), with medium fine blonde hair of average density.

Same patient after two procedures of Follicular Transplantation, spaced 11 months apart.

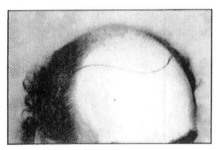

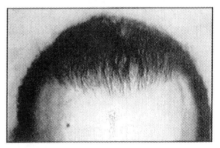

44-year-old male with extensive balding (Norwood Class 6), with slightly wavy dark hair of above average density.

Same patient after one procedure of Follicular Transplantation.

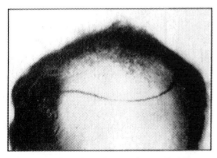

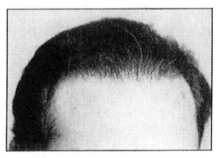

36-year-old male with moderate balding (Norwood Class 5a/6), with medium fine dark brown hair of high density.

Same patient after two procedures of Follicular Transplantation, spaced 9½ months apart.

Hair Replacement Successes

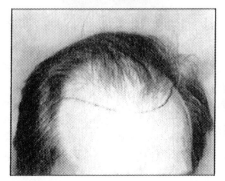

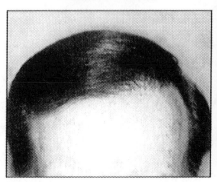

48-year-old male with thinning on top, but most balding limited to front (Norwood Class 5a), with medium weight brown hair.

Same patient after one procedure of Follicular Transplantation.

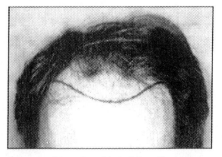

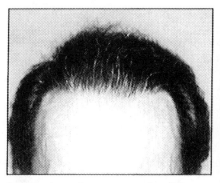

46-year-old male with balding limited to the front (Norwood Class 4a), with medium to coarse black hair.

Same patient after one procedure of Follicular Transplantation.

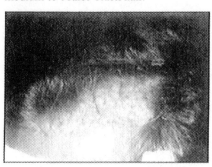

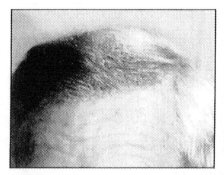

53-year-old male with old plugs that failed to grow hair. The visible white scars were produced by the hairless plugs.

Same patient after one repair procedure using Follicular Transplantation. After repair, the patient allowed hair to grow naturally gray.

Hair Replacement Casualties

The "Doll's Head" or "Pluggy Look" of old procedures that used large grafts. Unfortunately, many physicians still perform these types of disfiguring procedures.

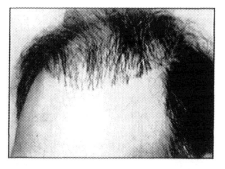

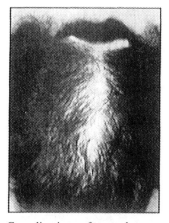

Complications of a poorly planned scalp reduction that produced a wide scar and a "Dog Ear" defect in the back of the scalp.

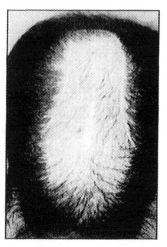

Configuration of a horseshoe-shaped scalp reduction with only the frontal rim of hair transplanted. The scalp reduction in this patient has significantly reduced the density of the donor area and increased the tightness of the scalp, limiting the amount of hair available to complete the transplant.

Toppik Successes

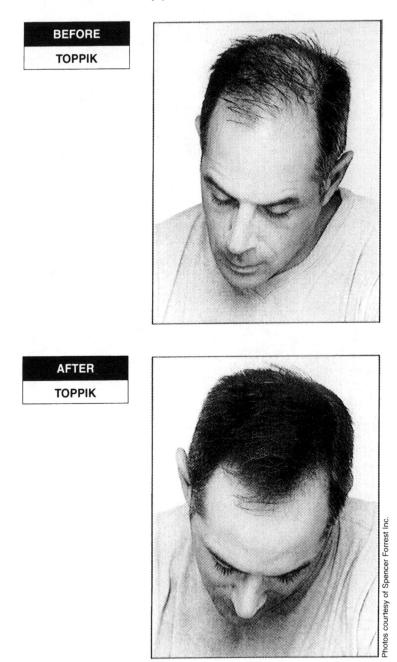

BEFORE
TOPPIK

AFTER
TOPPIK

Photos courtesy of Spencer Forrest Inc.

Toppik Successes

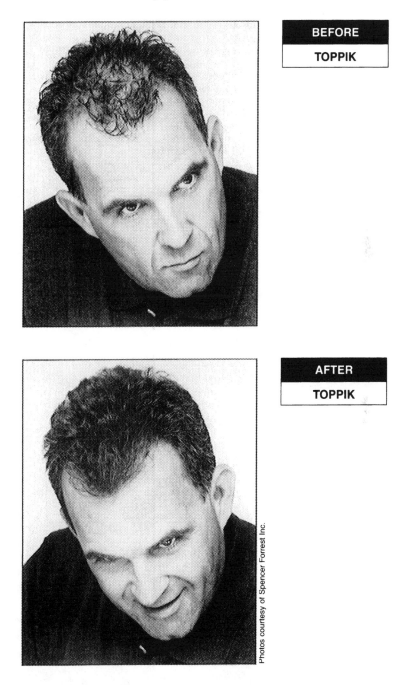

BEFORE

TOPPIK

AFTER

TOPPIK

Photos courtesy of Spencer Forrest Inc.

Toppik Successes

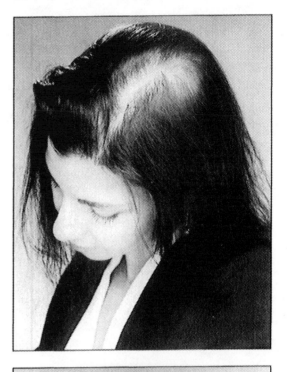

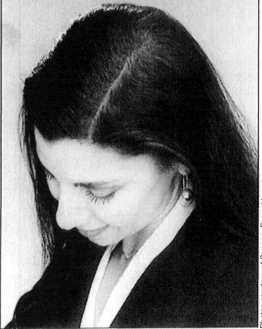

Photos courtesy of Spencer Forrest Inc.

to remove and reattach (every day), you still have tunnels on your head! If the tunnels are surgically removed, permanent scars are left on your scalp.

Sewing Hairpieces to the Scalp

Although this is illegal in every state in the United States, "in at least one state, New Jersey, some companies have been able to do this for years despite attempts by the New Jersey attorney general to put them permanently out of business," cautions esteemed surgeon William R. Rassman, M.D.

This is a barbaric procedure in which the hairpiece is actually sewn into your scalp. Since the stitches (sutures) aren't ever removed and don't dissolve—unlike in surgery, when they are either removed after the wound heals or they naturally dissolve—big problems ensue.

"Surgical sutures that are left in the skin for too long a time always cut through the skin just like the type of cheese knife that uses a wire as a cutting edge," says Rassman. "The sutures are always cutting their way out and have to be replaced."

This is further complicated by movement and pull, like touching and combing the hair, which tugs at the sutures.

Recurring infections and scarring result.

Wait, it gets worse. The scars "gradually cause almost total blockage of blood supply to the central portion of the scalp, and so the skin in the center of the scalp becomes replaced by a thin, parchmentlike layer of scar tissue," Rassman explains. "Any permanent hair that was present in the area surrounded by the suture is also destroyed. The damage is permanent."

About half a dozen years ago, while researching hair-replacement methods, I visited one of these companies in New Jersey. I was in a very early stage of hair loss and wasn't even yet a candidate for a hairpiece, let alone something as extreme and dangerous as sewing one onto my head. Nevertheless, the sales staff at this facility was relentless, trying to convince me that I needed their procedure. Of course, I was only there on a research mission, but I feel very sorry for anyone who was convinced to have this procedure.

Artificial Fibers Implanted in the Scalp

Imagine a crude version of hair transplantation, but instead of using your own donor hair, synthetic fibers are implanted in your head.

A man-made polymer called NIDO is used for these transplants. This form of nylon is implanted in small bundles directly into your scalp. Although this procedure is *not* done in the United States, it is most widely used in Japan and other countries, and many U.S. doctors have treated men who have shown up with disastrous effects from these implants they received in another country.

The fibers are shiny, artificial looking, and stiff. The texture doesn't look or feel like real hair. The implants cause chronic infections at the implant sites, and over time inflammation and infection can destroy the scalp.

Plugs of the scalp's natural oils (sebum) build up at the base of the fibers, and every few weeks the patient has to be treated to remove the sebum and to treat the ongoing infection.

As if this wasn't bad enough, the fibers are brittle and break easily. Styling and blow-drying cause them to frizz and become permanently damaged. Combing them can break them or pull them out. Infection can cause premature loss of natural hair follicles adjacent to the artificial fibers.

In short, this is like implanting fibers from your living-room carpet into your head, with severe consequences.

Hair Integration

A Paris-based company with U.S. headquarters in Beverly Hills and New York City offers a $20,000 (minimum!) procedure in which high-quality human hair is "integrated" with your own hair through a network of tiny, solid gold cylinders that attach the bought hair to your own hair.

Resembling a weave, this looks natural, but like every other weave it has tremendous drawbacks (see previous section on weaves), and to add insult to injury, maintenance on these integration systems can easily cost you $1,000 per month.

Both men and women have gotten excellent cosmetic results with this procedure, but the health concerns of a weave remain, although by using the cylinders, this kind of weave does allow for more breathing room between the attached hair, your own hair, and the scalp.

Buying a Hairpiece

If you want a weave or hairpiece that is bonded, the Hair Club for Men, though a bit pricey, does do an excellent job, but keep in mind the health disadvantages, as noted earlier in this chapter in the section about weaves.

If you're in the market for a traditional hairpiece, to be attached by clips or adhesive, you can buy one in your area by first asking the best hair salon in town to refer you to the best hairpiece studio in town, one whose work they have seen and think highly of.

At this studio, a small bit of your hair will be snipped off, so the makers of your hairpiece can match color, texture, density, and the like. The stylist will measure your scalp for a proper fitting.

The studio then orders your hairpiece from a wholesaler. They make this order based on the information you provide them concerning the quality of hairpiece you'd like to purchase.

When your hairpiece arrives at the studio, the stylist will custom fit it, trim it, and style it once it is attached to your head.

You may want to buy two hairpieces, so you have one to wear when the other one is out "in the shop." Hairpieces do need to be maintained, and you'll want to bring it to the studio you bought it from, or another one of your choosing, at least once a month for special cleaning, conditioning, and any repair or coloring that's needed.

6

COVER-UP PRODUCTS

All art is but imitation of nature.

—SENECA

Cover-up products can look quite natural, and many men use them with great success. In fact, you see men wearing these products all the time and don't even realize it. And I'm not referring to the guys on film and television, but to your colleagues, friends and neighbors.

How well these products work depends on which ones you use, the extent of your hair loss, and how you apply the products. They are easy to use and affordable—and no, they don't make a mess of you, your clothes or anyone else.

Let's take a look at the best cover-up products on the market today:

Toppik

If you have little or moderate hair loss, Toppik makes your hair look fuller, while still looking natural. Toppik is fibers made of keratin, the same protein human hair is made of. Thousands of these fibers come in a stylishly packaged jar, and to apply you gently shake the fibers directly from the container onto the thinning areas of your scalp. Using natural static electricity, these fibers attach to your existing hair, no matter how thin your hair strands may be.

Toppik is 99% organic keratin and 1% approved colorant, conditioners and glidants that keep the product flowing freely. It's considered safe to use with topical treatments, whether they're natural or pharmaceutical, and also safe to use if you are taking any natural or pharmaceutical treatments internally, such as saw palmetto or Propecia.

You can also use Toppik after hair transplants as soon as the recipient sites have healed. It's especially helpful after transplants while you're waiting for your new hair to grow out.

Although Toppik will not come out easily during daily wear, even in wind or rain, it does wash out easily and will not damage your hair or scalp. It won't brush out, so you can comb your hair and even run your fingers through it. Because Toppik washes out, it will also come out if you swim with your head underwater.

Toppik doesn't stain or streak, and you need not be concerned if some of the fibers land on your clothes. Just brush them right off.

Toppik comes in black, dark brown, medium brown, light brown, auburn, blonde, white and gray.

Couvre

Couvre Masking Lotion was the first cover-up product, and gained widespread use among theatrical make-up artists.

A scalp coloring product, Couvre is applied with a sponge applicator that comes in the package. Although it masks hair loss underneath some hair, you can't put it on bald spots unless there's a fair amount of hair covering them. It is ideal for thinning areas, no matter how large or small.

Couvre works visually by eliminating the contrast between your scalp and your hair, and since it also thickens the base of each hair, it does make hair appear thicker.

119

Although you can't use it on the edges of your hairline, you can use it all over the rest of your scalp under existing moderately thinning hair and it will look natural.

Couvre won't come off in the rain, you can swim with your head under water and it won't run or smear. The only way to remove Couvre is by shampooing it out.

You can apply Couvre to either dry or damp hair and scalp. It won't clog pores or interfere with hair growth, and once applied it takes about one minute to fully set.

Since Couvre's main ingredient is sesame oil, it's much like a tinted moisturizer. Couvre's color comes from iron oxides, which are naturally derived colorants that are approved for use around the face.

You can use Couvre even though you may be using a topical hair loss treatment. Just put Couvre on after the topical treatment has been completely absorbed.

Couvre comes in black, dark brown, medium brown, light brown, auburn, blonde, gray and white/gray.

Fullmore

Fullmore Colored Hair Thickener is a new product that acts like a Toppik and Couvre combination. Fullmore's spray applies tiny colored keratin fibers (the same ones used in Toppik) to your thinning hair and scalp.

Unlike the previous generation of spray cover-up products, Fullmore isn't messy and is very easy to control.

Fullmore comes in the same colors as Toppik: black, light black, dark brown, medium brown, light brown, auburn, blonde, white, and gray.

Fullmore's special polymers adhere to your own hair follicles, concealing bald spots and adding thickness to thin hair. After you apply it, wait 15–30 seconds and then apply any hair spray to seal it. Once sealed, it won't flake or come off until you shampoo.

These cover-up products can help you feel less self-conscious about your hair loss. You can use them alone, or in conjunction with hair loss treatments, and they work equally well for women as for men. To order the above-mentioned products or receive more information, call (800) 416-3325; or write: Spencer Forrest, Inc., 578 Post Road East, Westport, CT 06880; or visit the Web at www.regrow.com.

7

HAIR-LOSS TREATMENTS IN DEVELOPMENT

If you theorize too much, you can find
only the things that you understand. If
you do things beyond what you can
theorize about, you find something
that's a surprise.

—ROBERT CAVA

Even as Propecia, the breakthrough baldness prevention and treatment drug, was rolling through
the manufacturing process and out into pharmacies, scientists at Merck and other pharmaceutical
companies, as well as biotechnical companies,
universities, and labs around the world, were already working on the research, study, experi-
ments, and testing of plenty of other drugs and
treatments that will follow.

These new developments include using genes to cause hair follicles to grow hair, cloning your existing hair, and drugs specifically designed for women.

In this chapter, you'll find some of the most promising new preventions and treatments on the horizon. Some may be available before the decade is over, others are within five years of reaching the market, some are already available outside the United States and may soon be on the U.S. market, and still others are in early or intermediate stages of research and development.

Gene Therapy

Dr. Angela Christiano of Columbia University's Columbia-Presbyterian Medical Center in New York made history on January 30, 1998, when the journal *Science* published her discovery of the first human gene ever linked to hair loss.

The newly identified gene appears to play a critical role in the formation of hair.

This gene is not the one linked to androgenic alopecia—male pattern baldness—but to one particular rare form of alopecia, a condition in which people lose all of their hair.

This discovery, however, is a major breakthrough in the search for the gene that causes male pattern baldness as well as those genes that cause other strains of alopecia.

A San Diego biotech company, AntiCancer, Inc., was working on developing new diagnostic and therapeutic modalities for cancer when, much to their surprise, hair grew in an experiment regarding ways to grow cells.

Since they now had a way to cultivate hair-growing skin cells, they decided to pursue it. This led them to a breakthrough in the ability to deliver a gene's DNA coding directly to hair follicles. They are now working on identifying the genes involved in hair growth and hair loss so they can ultimately deliver those to the hair follicle.

Robert Hoffman, M.D., founder and president of AntiCancer, Inc., reported his findings in the journal *Nature Medicine* (July 1995).

The National Institutes of Health (NIH) is very encouraged by Hoffman's work.

"We have an enemy, hair follicle disease, and Dr. Hoffman has invented a 'gun' with which to fight that enemy," said Dr. Leonid B. Margolis, a researcher at the NIH. "He has demonstrated that the gun works by firing blanks at the hair follicles. What remains for us to do is to develop the ammunition that will make the gun useful in the fight against hair loss."

Dr. Hoffman notes that his gene-delivery process demonstrates "that genes can be targeted selectively to the most important cells of the hair follicle."

This work means that "highly selective, safe gene therapy for the hair process is feasible," he says.

Scientists at AntiCancer, Inc., have already developed a way to deliver melanin, which gives hair its color, to hair follicles.

Increasing the Hair's Growth Cycle with PTH

Initial research by Dr. Michael Holick of Boston University Medical School and researchers in Berlin shows that by blocking PTHrP, a chemical in the body that causes hair follicles to go into a resting cycle, hair follicles can return to their growth phase. Studies in mice show that scientists may have found the equivalent of the switch that turns inactive follicles back on. Human studies are scheduled to test the blocking agent, PTH.

More 5-Alpha-Reductase Inhibitors

By inhibiting the enzyme 5-alpha-reductase, finasteride at the 5 mg. dose in Merck's Proscar inhibits DHT production by 70 percent. In Merck's Propecia, the 1 mg. dose of finasteride inhibits DHT production by 60 percent. Scientists at Merck are working on more ways to inhibit the enzyme 5-alpha-reductase, which converts testosterone to hair-follicle-killing DHT. Drugs are in the research and development phase that work even faster than finasteride and can safely inhibit DHT production up to 98 percent.

Cyoctol

Upjohn, the pharmaceutical company that makes Rogaine (minoxidil), is studying and developing a new drug, cyoctol, that blocks the effects of testosterone on hair follicles. Initial studies show that 92 percent of the men in a one-year test showed some slowing of hair loss and some regrowth of hair. The drug is used externally, as a topical lotion applied to the head, and is still in the human-testing phase.

Aromatase

Scientists are researching aromatase, an enzyme that blocks or deactivates DHT's effect on hair follicles.

Dercos (Aminexil)

Developed by L'Oreal Pharmaceuticals in Paris, this drug is marketed in France for the treatment of women's androgenetic alopecia (the female version of male pattern baldness). Dercos is sold over-the-counter there and works by combating the hardening of the hair follicles, a hair-loss-causing condition prevalent among women with MPB.

RU 58841

The drug RU 58841, an androgen receptor blocker, inhibits the effects of testosterone and DHT, its derivative, on hair follicles. It is one of the most promising drugs in development, but it is currently caught in the middle of corporate politics and competition intrigue.

Nitroxide/TEMPOL

Baldness resulting from radiation affects many who undergo these treatments in cancer therapy as well as for other conditions.

The Radiation Oncology Branch of the National Cancer Institute is studying the effects of topically applying the compound nitroxide radical TEMPOL to the scalp, in an effort to prevent radiation-induced baldness. Initial studies are promising.

Cloning

Scientists are at work on cloning human hair, so that perhaps in the near future you can donate to yourself all of the hair you'll need regardless of how much "donor hair" is growing in your donor sites. By cloning *one* of your hairs, scientists will be able to make as many as are needed to completely fill in all your balding areas.

Dr. Colin Jahoda, of the University of Durham in England, is the world's leading authority on hair cloning, and has already grown a cloned hair on his arm. Research is also ongoing at the University of Washington in Seattle, in the Netherlands, and in Korea.

Dutasteride

A dual 5-alpha reductase inhibitor, this drug developed by Glaxo Wellcome inhibits Type I and

II of the enzyme (Propecia only inhibits Type II), and early testing shows it can be more potent than Propecia. It is expected to be FDA-approved for prostate treatment by 2001, and for hair loss by 2003.

APPENDIXES

Babies haven't any hair,
Old men's heads are just as bare;
Between the cradle and the grave
Lies a haircut and a shave.
         —SAMUEL HOFFENSTEIN, *Songs of*
         Faith in the Year after Next

How's It Growing: Hair Basics

Your hair is dead. It's always been dead. It's always going to be dead. That's okay, it's supposed to be. While hair follicles are very much alive, at least until DHT shrinks them to death in those who are balding, hair itself is actually composed of dead cells that grow out of the follicles.

Hair follicles are tiny pockets of live, dividing cells just under the skin. These hair follicles are fed by blood vessels that lead into them and by oil glands within the follicles. These oil glands make your hair shine too.

Hair is made of a protein called *keratin,* which also hardens the hair.

"Synthesis of proteins requires a great investment of energy," explains William R. Rassman, M.D. "When a person becomes ill or malnourished, the hair stops growing; when the illness or malnutrition is severe or prolonged, the hair will even fall out. When hair begins to grow back, that's an early sign that recovery has begun."

Keratin is the same protein that hardens nails, which is why nails can also be affected by illness.

Each strand of hair consists of three layers: The outer layer is called the *cuticle,* the middle layer is called the *cortex,* and the inner layer is called the *medulla.*

The *cuticle* is thin and has no color, and its job is to protect the thicker cortex, which contains melanin, the pigment that colors your hair. There are only two kinds of melanin: *eumelanin* makes your hair black or brown, depending on how much of it your cells pack into each hair. *Pheomelanin* makes your hair red.

Blond hair contains very little melanin. Melanin is produced by *melanocytes,* and when they can no longer produce as much melanin as is needed to keep the hairs colored, because the *tyrosinase* enzymes that create melanin are lost, hair will turn gray and eventually white. Not only age but stress and physical illness can accelerate the graying process.

Human hair is classified into two main types: *Vellus* hair is fine and can range from what we call peach fuzz to hairs that are so fine they are almost invisible except upon very close or microscopic inspection. *Terminal* hair is the coarser, longer, more visible hair.

Except for the palms of the hands and the soles of the feet, most of the human body is covered with hair.

The shape of the *cortex* in cross section determines whether hair will be straight, wavy, or curly. The cross section of the cortex is cylindrical in straight hair and oval in curly hair. Slight variations in these shapes determine variations in straightness, waviness, and curliness.

The innermost layer of each strand of hair, the *medulla,* reflects light and therefore gives hair its color tones.

Like so many other aspects of your body, most of your hair's qualities are controlled by heredity.

GROWTH CYCLES

The average head has 100,000 hair follicles, and they are not all in the same growth phase at the same time.

Hair usually grows about half an inch each month. Each strand will grow at this pace for about two years. Then it rests for a while and eventually falls out, to be replaced by another strand about to break the surface of your scalp. At any given time, 90 percent of your hairs are in the growing phase.

Normal hair loss in this cycle is between fifty to a hundred strands per day. If you don't have male pattern baldness, or another balding condition, the hair you find in your brush or comb, on the bathroom floor, in the bathtub drain, or anywhere else is completely normal.

Normally, hair falls out and is replaced at staggered intervals, from follicles all over your head, so that this natural, cyclical hair loss is never noticed on your head. You won't lose just front, top, side, or back hair at the end of a cycle; hair is falling out at various times from all parts of your head.

You may be surprised to learn that even with extensive male pattern baldness, you lose only 30 to 40 percent of your hair. It only looks like more because most of the hair loss is on the front and top of your head. (See Norwood Scale on page 135.)

HORMONES AND HAIR QUALITY

As noted earlier in this chapter and in Chapters One and Two, your health and nutrition play a

Norwood Classifications
Male Pattern Baldness • Main Classes

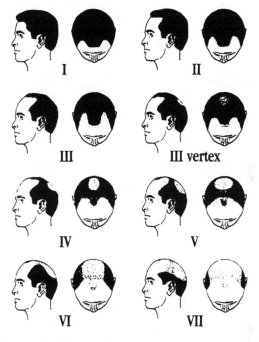

Male Pattern Baldness • Type "A" Variants

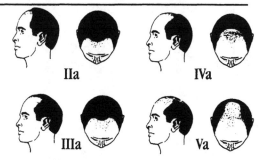

Permission to reprint given by O'Tar Norwood.

vital role in your ability to grow and keep hair, as well as the quality of your hair. Hormones in particular have a profound effect on hair, as detailed in Chapters One, Two, and Three, but hormones' effects are not limited to male pattern baldness.

Hormonal changes can also make hair more oily: Higher levels of hormones mean higher levels of oil in the hair follicles' oil glands.

For women, the drastic hormonal changes of pregnancy can cause hair to become more oily and can even change hair from curly to straight. Sometimes the change in curliness is permanent.

After pregnancy, and also during menopause, hormonal decreases can cause mild hair loss. Usually, once hormone levels return to normal, within a few months after childbirth, hair will return to its normal volume. During menopause, women who replenish lost hormones or boost low hormone levels through natural methods or by taking synthetic estrogen and progesterone drugs can also increase the volume of their hair.

Women taking birth-control pills may also experience similar hormone-induced changes in their hair.

CARING FOR YOUR HAIR

So much of what we do in the name of style ends up hurting our hair.

Hair can be split or damaged by excessive or harsh brushing, exposure to sun, wind, and chlorine, and even by hairstyles that pull hair too tightly on a regular basis. How you brush or comb your hair is important to its health. Start at the scalp and work down to the ends to ensure that the oil from the follicles will be distributed completely down the length of each strand. Back-combing or teasing hair can split or damage it, and prevents it from receiving the much-needed oil that would be spread by regular combing or brushing.

Split ends can appear in the middle of a strand when it's damaged and at the tip of an older strand. Trimming the tips will eliminate the split ends. If you wear your hair short, those frequent haircuts mean that you will probably never have a split hair tip.

Hair sprays, gels, mousses, and other styling preparations often contain alcohol and other chemicals that can dry out and damage hair. Products with natural ingredients are healthier for your hair.

Hair conditioners moisturize and add protein to the hair shaft, but they don't penetrate to the interior portions of the hair. Conditioners can protect and strengthen hair by keeping it supple and therefore less likely to split from brushing or styling. Hot-oil treatments merely coat the hair, making it softer and shinier, but they do not moisturize the hair.

Moisture is essential to healthy hair. When you shampoo, your hair receives moisture from the water, and if you have naturally dry hair you can also use a shampoo containing moisturizers, specially formulated for dry hair. Those two-in-one shampoos that are also conditioners may be too heavy and slick, so use a separate shampoo and a separate conditioner no matter what type of hair you have.

If you don't shampoo often enough, dirt, oils, styling products, and the residue from pollution, smoke, and just everyday life will build up, clog your hair follicles, prevent nutrients from reaching your scalp and hair, and eventually prevent it from growing properly.

Wet hair is easy to stretch so it is also easily damaged. Untangle wet hair with your fingers or a wide-toothed comb, not a brush.

If your hair is oily or short, shampoo it every day. If it's longer and normal or dry, you can wash it every two days. Always use conditioner after shampooing.

Permanents to wave or curl hair, and processes to straighten it, work by using chemicals that unlock particular molecular links in the hair strands, followed by other chemicals that relock them into different arrangements. These chemicals can not only damage hair, but, if not used properly or if used too often, they can also cause your hair to fall out. The hair will grow back unless there has been severe follicle damage, which is very rare.

BODY HAIR

Different kinds of hair grow on various parts of the body. "Although most terminal hairs may appear to be similar," says. Dr. Rassman, "there are really several distinct subtypes." And these hairs also grow and fall out in cycles.

Eyelash and nose hairs are called *cilia,* and they are different from head and body hairs. Pubic and underarm hairs are also very different from terminal head hairs.

"These diverse types of hair can be distinguished from each other by the lengths to which they grow and characteristics such as texture and tendency to curl," says Dr. Rassman.

These body hairs may also gray as you age, though usually more slowly than the hair on your head and on a man's beard.

GENERAL HAIR LOSS

Hair loss from illness, radiation, or chemotherapy can occur not only on the head but on other parts of the body too. This hair loss is usually temporary, but it can be permanent.

The condition known as *alopecia areata* should not be confused with male pattern baldness or baldness resulting from other conditions, situations, or medications. *Alopecia areata* is thought to be an immune-system disorder in which the body's defense forces mistakenly target hair follicles as if they were foreign invaders, like bacteria or viruses. This kind of baldness is most often temporary and periodic, but it can be permanent. It is characterized by patches of baldness on the heads of both men and women (and on men's beards), and can range from mild, with just a few bald areas, to severe, resulting in complete baldness. Sometimes all body hair is lost as well. This is the result of *alopecia totalis.*

Alopecia can also be triggered by stress and is seen most commonly in young adults.

EXCESSIVE HAIR GROWTH

On the other end of the spectrum, excessive hair is called *hirsutism,* and those with it are medically classified as *hirsute.*

While excessive hairiness of the entire body or particular areas can be genetic, it can also be caused by hormonal imbalances in men and women, which can be triggered by a number of factors, including overactive adrenal glands, ovarian cysts or tumors (in women), adrenal tumors, thyroid gland disorders, pituitary gland disorders, and the use of drugs such as steroids, birth-control pills, estrogen, progesterone, testosterone, and others that contain hormones or affect hormonal balance. The treatment for hirsutism is based on treating its cause. Even after successful treatment of the cause, or ceasing to take the drugs that are causing hirsutism, excessive hair growth may not diminish entirely. Hair-removal treatments can then be considered, including the newest laser and laser electrolysis technology, regular electrolysis (destruction of the hair follicle with an electric current), waxing, shaving, tweezing, and using depilatories that dissolve hair. Finasteride is also being tested for use in this disorder.

Busting Hair-Loss Myths

MYTH: Male pattern baldness is inherited from your mother's side of the family.

FACT: The gene for male pattern baldness can come from your mother's or your father's gene pool; therefore, baldness can be inherited from either side of the family.

◆

MYTH: Losing an average of a hundred hairs per day is nothing to worry about because it's normal.

FACT: If you don't have male pattern baldness, that's true, because the hairs that fall out will soon be replaced by new hairs sprouting from the hair follicles underneath the skin. If you *do* have male pattern baldness, however, even losing the "normal" hundred hairs a day can be a concern because many of those hairs are being shed by follicles that are in the process of dying, and therefore the new hairs those follicles make will be progressively thinner until the follicles are only capable of making fine, "peach fuzz" hairs. Eventually those follicles will die and no longer produce any hairs at all.

◆

MYTH: You can increase the number of hair follicles by drugs, natural or chemical treatments, massage, diet, or other means.

FACT: No. The number and diameter of your hair follicles is completely out of your control—it's hereditary. Nothing you do will alter how many hair follicles you have. But you can use preventive and treatment measures outlined in this book to combat the follicle-killing effects of DHT, the androgen created when the hormone testosterone is acted upon by the enzyme 5-alpha-reductase.

◆

MYTH: Cutting your hair can make it grow back faster and thicker.

FACT: No. Hair grows at an average rate of half an inch per month. Because each hair shaft is slightly thicker at its base compared to its tip, hair can temporarily *appear* thicker for about a week after it has been significantly cut. But cutting hair has absolutely *no* effect on each strand's thickness or on the number of hairs that will sprout from follicles.

◆

MYTH: If left uncut, my hair will just keep growing and growing.

FACT: No. Length depends on your hair's natural cycle, which is unique to *you.* The longer the hair's growth phase, the longer the hair will grow. If you have a naturally long growth phase, you can grow your hair to well below your waist. If you have a naturally shorter growth phase, your hair will be shed before it grows that long and only grow to a certain length. The duration of your particular growth phase is based on heredity and is affected by nutrition.

◆

MYTH: Wearing a hat causes hair loss.

FACT: As long as you don't regularly wear a hat that's so tight that it restricts circulation—blood flow to the hair follicles—this will not cause hair loss. It can, however, damage hair because of the effects of sweat, dirt, and skin particles that can clog pores.

◆

MYTH: Blow-drying can cause hair loss.

FACT: No. But it can dry, burn, and damage hair that may then fall out, to be replaced by new hair that will sprout from the follicle beneath the skin during the growth phase.

Hair Loss as a Side Effect of Prescription Drugs

Many routinely prescribed prescription drugs can cause temporary hair loss, exacerbate male pattern baldness, trigger its onset, or cause permanent hair loss. The drugs on the following list do *not* include those used in chemotherapy and radiation for the treatment of cancer.

If your doctor prescribes any of the following drugs, ask if one that does *not* have hair loss as a possible side effect can be substituted. You may also want to look into the possibility of using an effective natural treatment instead of a prescription drug, and you can discuss this with your doctor and naturopathic physician or health-care practitioner.

The brand names of the drugs are listed first, followed by the drug's generic name in parentheses. The drugs are listed by category, according to the conditions they treat. In some categories, individual drugs are not listed, and you will want to discuss the possibility of hair loss as a side effect of using drugs that treat that particular condition, since many of them *do* contribute to hair loss.

ACNE

- All drugs derived from vitamin A as treatments for acne or other conditions, including:
  - Accutane *(isotretinoin)*

BLOOD

- Anticoagulants (blood thinners), including:
  - Panwarfin ⎫
  - Sofarin ⎬ *(warfarin sodium)*
  - Coumadin ⎭
  - Heparin injections

CHOLESTEROL

- Cholesterol-lowering drugs, including:
  - Atronid-S *(clofibrate)*
  - Lopid *(gemfibrozil)*

CONVULSIONS/EPILEPSY

- Anticonvulsants, including:
  - Tridone *(trimethadione)*

DEPRESSION

- Antidepression drugs, including:
  - Prozac *(fluoxetine hydrochloride)*
  - Zoloft *(sertraline hydrochloride)*
  - Paxil *(paroxetine)*
  - Anafranil *(clomipramine)*
  - Janimine ⎫
  - Tofranil ⎬ *(imipramine)*
  - Tofranil PM ⎭
  - Adapin ⎫ *(doxepin)*
  - Sinequan ⎭
  - Surmontil *(trimipramine)*
  - Pamelor ⎫ *(nortriptyline)*
  - Ventyl ⎭
  - Elavin ⎫ *(amitriptyline)*
  - Endep ⎭
  - Norpramin ⎫ *(desipramine)*
  - Pertofrane ⎭

- Vivactil *(protriptyline hydrochloride)*
- Asendin *(amoxapine)*
- Haldol *(haloperidol)*

DIET

- Amphetamines

FUNGUS

- Antifungals

GLAUCOMA

- The beta-blocker drugs, including:
  - Timoptic Eye Drops ⎫
  - Timoptic Ocudose ⎬ *(timolol)*
  - Timoptic XC ⎭

GOUT

- Lopurin ⎫ (allopurinol)
- Zyloprim ⎭

HEART

- Many drugs prescribed for the heart, including those known as the beta blockers, which are also used to treat high blood pressure, and include:

- Tenormin *(atenolol)*
- Lopressor *(metoprolol)*
- Corgard *(nadolol)*
- Inderal and Inderal LA *(propanolol)*
- Blocadren *(timolol)*

HIGH BLOOD PRESSURE

- See above list of beta blockers under "Heart."

HORMONAL CONDITIONS

- All hormone-containing drugs and drugs prescribed for hormone-related, reproductive, male-specific, and female-specific conditions and situations have the potential to cause hair loss, including:
- Birth-control pills
- Hormone-replacement therapy (HRT) for women (estrogen or progesterone)
- Male androgenic hormones and all forms of testosterone
- Anabolic steroids
- Prednisone and other steroids

INFLAMMATION

- Many anti-inflammatory drugs, including those prescribed for localized pain, swelling, and injury.

- Arthritis drugs
- Nonsteroidal Anti-Inflammatory Drugs (NSAIDS), including:
  - Naprosyn ⎫
  - Anaprox ⎬ *(naproxen)*
  - Anaprox DS ⎭
  - Indocin ⎫ *(indomethacin)*
  - Indocin SR ⎭
  - Clinoril *(sulindac)*
- An anti-inflammatory that is also used as a chemotherapy drug:
  - Methotrexate (MTX) ⎫
  - Rheumatex ⎬ *(methotrexate)*
  - Folex ⎭

PARKINSON'S DISEASE

- Levadopa/L-dopa *(dopar, larodopa)*

STOMACH (see "Ulcer" below)

THYROID DISORDERS

- Many of the drugs used to treat the thyroid.

ULCER

- Many of the drugs used to treat indigestion, stomach difficulties, and ulcers, including over-the-counter dosages and prescription dosages.

149

- Tagamet *(cimetidine)*
- Zantac *(ranitidine)*
- Pepcid *(famotidine)*

A Note to Women

Women cannot use the same treatment or preventive measures as men when treating androgenetic alopecia (male pattern baldness).

Unless you are beyond childbearing age, or are unable to get pregnant, you will not even begin to consider using the drugs that men can use to treat MPB. In some circumstances, your doctor may prescribe Propecia or other treatments used by men, but only if you will not be getting pregnant or carrying a pregnancy to full term.

Propecia's active agent, finasteride, can cause birth defects in male fetuses.

As with the pharmaceutical drugs that treat MPB, the herbal treatments are only intended generally for men. Do *not* use them if you will be getting pregnant. The DHT-inhibiting abilities of these herbs can affect the fetus.

Discuss all of this with your physician before determining your course of treatment.

Take heart, as scientists *are* at work developing potential treatments for women who suffer from hair loss.

Women have also had great success with hair transplantation. It is highly recommended for some women with androgenetic alopecia.

You should also seek to determine the origin of your hair loss by having a complete physical, including tests to determine your hormone levels and any conditions that may be causing a hormonal imbalance that could be the catalyst for your hair loss.

Hair-Loss Styling Tips

There are several easy ways to make fine or thinning hair appear fuller, or transplanted hair appear fuller:

- Use thickening shampoos, which add body and improve texture.
- Condition your hair *before* you shampoo. This allows you to get all the benefits of conditioning without it weighing down or flattening your hair.
- Shampoo daily. You only need to wash your hair once during this process. There's no need to reapply the shampoo for a second washing, as this can dry out your hair.
- Use a blow-dryer at a low setting. This will

add volume to your hair and help direct it for styling.

- *Do not mousse or gel your hair.* This makes hair appear thinner by weighing it down.
- Use a good hairspray or finishing spray instead of mousses and gels. After drying hair completely, lightly mist it with spray, let dry, comb through, style as desired, then spray again. This will make your hair look very full while keeping it under control.
- If your hair is thinning or sparse in front, lightening or highlighting the front will make the thinning area less noticeable, especially if you have a naturally high contrast between your skin and hair color. This contrast is reduced by the highlighting. This is *not* advised for those with dark skin and dark hair, however.

Hair-Replacement Products by Mail Order

Many of the high-quality hair systems costing thousands of dollars can be purchased by mail order. It is possible to get high-quality units at half the price of those purchased at hair studios. Also available are all of the attachment products, including bonding agents, adhesive removers, clips, and anything else you might need. I personally think this is the way to go. It is easy, fast, and private. You can then bring the piece to any studio to have it attached and styled.

Anthony Hair Salon
445 Park Avenue
New York, N.Y. 10022
(212) 759-2340
(212) 688-4932

RESOURCES

Recommended Reading

BOOKS

- Antol, Marie Nadine. *Healing Teas: A Practical Guide to the Medicinal Teas of the World.* Garden City Park, NY: Avery, 1996.
- Benson, Herbert, M.D. *Timeless Healing.* New York: Scribner, 1996.
- Brown, Don J. *Herbal Prescriptions for Better Health.* Rocklin, CA: Prima Publishing, 1996.
- Chopra, Deepak, M.D. *Ageless Body, Timeless Mind.* New York: Harmony Books, 1993.
- Diamond, Nina L. *Purify Your Body: Natural Remedies for Detoxing from 50 Everyday Situations.* New York: Crown, 1997.
- Kimbrall, Andrew. *The Masculine Mystique.* New York: Ballantine, 1995.
- Pizzorno, Joe, N.D. *Total Wellness.* Rocklin, CA: Prima Publishing, 1996.

- Pizzorno, Joe, N.D., and Michael Murray, N.D. *Encyclopedia of Natural Medicine.* Rocklin, CA: Prima Publishing, 1991.
- Robbins, John. *Diet for a New America.* Walpole, NH: Stillpoint Publishing, 1997.
- Robbins, John. *Reclaiming Our Health.* Tiburon, CA: H.J. Kramer, 1996.
- Sears, Barry, Ph.D., *The Zone.* New York: Regan Books, 1995.
- Somer, Elizabeth. *The Essential Guide to Vitamins and Minerals.* New York: HarperCollins, 1995.
- Weill, Andrew, M.D. *Health and Healing* (rev. ed.). New York: Houghton Mifflin, 1995.
- Weill, Andrew, M.D. *Natural Health, Natural Medicine* (rev. ed.). New York: Houghton Mifflin, 1995.
- Weill, Andrew, M.D. *Spontaneous Healing.* New York: Knopf, 1995.

BOOKS FOR WOMEN

- Blum, Jeanne Elizabeth. *Woman Heal Thyself.* Boston: Charles E. Tuttle, 1995.
- Carlson, Karen J., M.D., Stephanie A. Eisenstat, M.D., and Terra Ziporyn, Ph.D. *The Harvard Guide to Women's Health.* Cambridge: Harvard University Press, 1995.
- Elias, Jason, and Katherine Ketchum. *In the*

House of the Moon. New York: Warner Books, 1995.

- Gladstar, Rosemary. *Herbal Healing for Women.* New York: Simon & Schuster, 1993.
- Healy, Bernadine, M.D. *A New Prescription for Women's Health.* New York: Penguin, 1996.
- Horrigan, Bonnie J. *Red Moon Passage.* New York: Harmony Books, 1996.
- Hutchinson, Karen Anne, M.D. *What Every Woman Needs to Know about Estrogen.* New York: Plume, 1997.
- Kobren, Spencer, *The Truth About Women's Hair Loss.* Chicago: Contemporary Books, 2000.
- Lonsdorf, N., and M. Lonsdorf. *A Woman's Best Medicine.* New York: Tarcher/Putnam, 1993.
- Mass, Brown, and Bruning. *The Mend Clinic Guide to Natural Medicine for Menopause and Beyond.* New York: Dell, 1997.
- Murray, M. *Natural Alternatives to Over-the-Counter Prescription Drugs.* New York: William Morrow, 1994.
- Northrup, Christiane, M.D. *Women's Bodies, Women's Wisdom.* New York: Bantam Books, 1994.
- Ojeda, Linda, Ph.D. *Menopause without Medicine* (3rd ed.). Alameda, CA: Hunter House, 1995.

PUBLICATIONS

Natural Health
P.O. Box 7440
Red Oak, IA 51591
(800) 526-8440

> Subscription address and phone number. Bimonthly magazine.

HerbalGram, Journal of the American Botanical Council and the Herbal Research Foundation
(512) 331-8868

> The Botanical Council has a bookstore too. For information and orders, call (800) 373-7105.

Dermatologic Surgery (medical journal)
930 North Meacham Road
Schaumburg, IL 60173
(847) 330-9830

International Journal of Aesthetic & Restorative Surgery (medical journal)
c/o George Faber, M.D., Secretary
200 West Esplanade Avenue, Suite 102
Kenner, LA 70065
(504) 471-3130

Organizations

The list below does *not* include any of the medical associations among whose members are doctors who perform hair-transplantation surgery or any of the trade associations in the hair-loss "industry."

This omission is entirely intentional because those associations will recommend members who may still be performing outdated procedures that can be harmful and can leave the patient with aesthetically unacceptable results.

For a list of recommended physicians who perform follicular transplantation, see that section in this Resource Guide.

The organizations listed below can provide you with information you may need in your all-inclusive hair-loss prevention and treatment efforts.

National Institutes of Health (NIH)
OAM Public Information Center
Office of Alternative Medicine (OAM)
Suite 450
6120 Executive Blvd.
Rockville, MD 20892
(301) 402-2466

The NIH is a government agency that funds and coordinates research and clinical studies into *all* areas of health and medicine, including alternative or natural medicine. The OAM can also refer you to other departments regarding pharmaceutical studies and other areas.

American Association of Naturopathic Physicians
2366 Eastlake Ave. East
Suite 322
Seattle, WA 98102
(206) 328-8510

American Herbalists Guild
Box 1683
Soquel, CA 95073
(408) 464-2441

Herb Research Foundation
1007 Pearl Street, #200
Boulder, CO 80302
(303) 440-2265

American Holistic Medical Association
4101 Lake Boone Trail, #201
Raleigh, NC 27607
(919) 787-5146

Association of Natural Medicine Pharmacists
(707) 887-1351

> Provides pharmacists with up-to-date scientific information on natural medicines.

Merck & Co.
Box 4
West Point, PA 19486
(215) 652-5000

Merck is the pharmaceutical company that manufactures both Propecia and Proscar.

Pharmacia & Upjohn
100 Route 206 North
Peapack, NJ 07977
(908) 901-8000

Pharmacia & Upjohn is the pharmaceutical company that manufactures Rogaine.

National Alopecia Areata Foundation
P.O. Box 150760
San Rafael, CA 94915
(415) 456-4274

Women's Health

Women to Women/Christiane Northrup, M.D.
One Pleasant Street
Yarmouth, ME 04096
(207) 846-6163

Women's International Pharmacy
(800) 279-5708

Prescription drugs and natural medicines can
be ordered by your physician.

National Alopecia Areata Foundation
(see listing under Organizations in this Resource
Guide)

National Women's Health Resource Center
Suite 325
2440 M Street N.W.
Washington, D.C. 10037
(202) 293-6045

National Black Women's Health Project
1237 Ralph Abernathy Blvd. S.W.
Atlanta, GA 30310
(800) 275-2947

National Latina Health Organization
P.O. Box 7567
Oakland, CA 94601
(510) 534-1362

National Women's Health Network
514 10th Street N.W.
Washington, D.C. 20004
(202) 347-1140

Herbal and Natural Products

Herbal and natural products can be ordered directly from the following:

Organic Planet
430 W. 24th Street, #1-D
New York, NY 10011
(800) 627-3631

Mountain Rose Herbs
(800) 879-3337

Sage Mountain Herbal Center
Box 420
East Barre, VT 05649
(902) 479-9825

Mountain Ark Trading Co.
120 South East Avenue
Fayetteville, AR 72701
(800) 643-8909

Herb Products Co.
11012 Magnolia Blvd.
North Hollywood, CA 81601

Frontier Direct
Box 127
Norway, IA 52318
(800) 726-5404

Gold Mine Natural Food Co.
1947 30th Street
San Diego, CA 92102
(800) 475-2000

Web Sites

These Web sites can offer the most comprehensive information regarding hair loss, and can also link you to many other pertinent sites on the Internet:

- *www.thebald.truth.org* (the author's Web site)
- *www.keratin.com*
- *www.hairtoday.com*
- *www.regrow.com*
- *www.regrowth.com*
- *www.hairsite.com*
- *www.hairboutique.com*

Guide to Physicians for Hair Transplantation

The physicians in this guide perform state-of-the-art follicular transplantation and are recognized by their peers as leaders in the field, not only for their medical expertise but for their active role in educating their fellow physicians (as well as patients) in the most recent and welcome innovations in hair-transplantation surgery. These physicians do regular research, publish in medical journals, present research findings and techniques at medical conferences, and are vocal advocates for continued change in the field.

Because an excellent physician skilled at follicular transplantation may not be located in your city or even your state, you may want to keep in mind that many patients travel for their transplantation procedure, which is done in one day at the doctor's medical office.

This guide is presented in alphabetical order.

Michael Beehner, M.D.
10 Railroad Place, #102
Saratoga Springs, NY 12866
(518) 581-1872

- Surgeon/Board Certified by the American Board of Hair Restoration Surgery
- Family Medicine/Board Certified by the American Board of Family Practice
- Associate Clinical Professor of Medicine at Albany Medical Center, Albany, NY

Dr. Beehner was among the first forty physicians in the United States to become certified by the new American Board of Hair Restoration Surgery.

He graduated from Loyola University in 1967, then received his doctor of medicine degree from the University of Illinois Medical School in 1971.

Dr. Beehner interned in family practice from 1971 to 1972 at Wesley Medical Center in Wichita, Kansas.

He did his residency in general surgery from 1974 to 1975 at St. Francis Medical Center in Wichita, Kansas, and then had a residency in Family Practice from 1975 to 1977 at the University of Wisconsin.

Dr. Beehner was also with the U.S. Public Health Service's National Health Service Corps, stationed in West Winfield, New York, from 1972 to 1974, between his internship and his first residency.

Dr. Beehner is active in a number of professional societies and has served as president of medical staff at Moses-Ludington Hospital in Ticonderoga, New York, and as president of the Essex County Medical Society.

He has been active in hair-transplant surgery research and clinical presentations. His publications include "The Frontal Forelock Concept in Hair Replacement Surgery" in the *American Journal of Cosmetic Surgery* (1997) and "A Frontal Forelock/Central Density Framework for Hair

Transplantation" in *Dermatologic Surgery Journal* (1997); his work has also appeared in *International Hair Transplant Forum.*

He has lectured and performed live surgery at the Annual Live Surgery Workshop and presented lectures at the annual meeting of the International Society of Hair Replacement Surgery. He is the 1995 recipient of the Outstanding Achievement Award presented by the American Academy of Facial Plastic and Reconstructive Surgery.

Robert M. Bernstein, M.D.
125 East 63rd Street
New York, NY 10021
(212) 872-1461

- Dermatologist/Board Certified in Dermatology/Fellow of the American Academy of Dermatology
- Assistant Clinical Professor of Dermatology at the College of Physicians and Surgeons of Columbia University in New York City
- Associate in the Dermatology Service, Columbia-Presbyterian Medical Center, New York City, where he teaches dermatologic and laser surgery and hair transplantation

Serving as chief resident, Dr. Bernstein received his dermatologic training at the Albert Einstein College of Medicine in New York. He graduated cum laude from Tulane University, achieving the status of Tulane scholar. He received his doctor of medicine degree at the University of Medicine and Dentistry of New Jersey and was the recipient of the Dr. Jacob Bleiberg Award for Excellence in Dermatology.

His contributions to the field of hair transplantation have earned Dr. Bernstein the honor of "Surgeon of the Month" in *Hair Transplant Forum International.* He first introduced the technique of follicular transplantation in the *International Journal of Aesthetic and Restorative Surgery* and at the International Society of Hair Restoration Surgery (see Chapter Four). He regularly speaks at medical society conferences.

Dr. Bernstein's recently published articles include: "Follicular Transplantation: Patient Evaluation and Surgical Planning," "Are Scalp Reductions Still Indicated?," "Laser Hair Transplantation: Is It Really State of the Art?," and "The Aesthetics of Follicular Transplantation."

Roy Jones, M.D.
1840 Mesquite Ave.
Suite D
Lake Havasu City, AZ 86403
(520) 855-3077

- Surgeon/Board Certified by the American Board of Surgery

Dr. Jones graduated from Wichita State University in 1970. He received his doctor of medicine degree from the University of Kansas School of Medicine in 1974.

He did a combined rotating internship and general surgery residency at the University of Kansas in Wichita from 1974 to 1979. He has served as chief of surgery at Wurtsmith Air Force Base hospital in Michigan and has been the vice chairman of the Nevada State Emergency Medical System's Trauma Task Force.

He has served on the American College of Surgeons' Committee on Trauma and has been an advanced trauma life-support instructor.

Dr. Jones is active in professional societies, encouraging the advancement of hair-transplantation surgery.

Robert Blaine Lehr, M.D.
5701 N. Portland, #310
Oklahoma City, OK 73112
(405) 951-4970

- Dermatologist/Board Certified by the American Board of Dermatology

Dr. Lehr is an associate of O'Tar Norwood, M.D., (see Norwood entry on page 172) joining Dr. Norwood's practice in 1995.

Dr. Lehr graduated from the University of

Oklahoma in 1986 with honors. At the university's College of Medicine, he received numerous awards, including the Tom Lowry Award for ranking first in the class after his first year, and the Mark R. Everett Award for most promise as a second-year student. He received his doctor of medicine degree from the University of Oklahoma College of Medicine in 1990.

He interned at Baptist Medical Center in Oklahoma City from 1990 to 1991, then did his dermatology residency at the University of Oklahoma from 1992 to 1995.

He is a member of a number of professional societies and publishes frequently in *Hair Transplant Forum International.*

Bobby L. Limmer, M.D.
14615 San Pedro Ave., Suite 210
One Medical Park
San Antonio, TX 78232
(210) 496-9929

- Dermatologist/Board Certified by the American Board of Dermatology

Dr. Limmer introduced the use of the microscope into the hair-transplantation procedure (see Chapter Four) and has been at the leading edge of transplantation-surgery innovations, giving more than thirty presentations at prestigious medical conferences and publishing more than a dozen articles in leading medical journals, including *Dermatologic Surgery, Advances in Dermatology, Dermatologic Surgery and Oncology,* and in *Hair Transplant Forum International.*

He graduated magna cum laude from Texas A&M University in 1964. He received his doctor of medicine degree from the University of Texas, Galveston, in 1968.

Dr. Limmer interned at Fitzsimons General Hospital in Denver from 1968 to 1969 and did his residency in dermatology at Brooke Army Medical Center in San Antonio, Texas, from 1969 to 1972.

He served in the U.S. Army Medical Corps from 1966 to 1974, receiving a U.S. Army Commendation Medal.

Dr. Limmer has had many academic appointments and fellowships and has been a clinical professor at the University of Texas Health Center in San Antonio. He is very active in professional societies and has held a number of offices, including president of the San Antonio Dermatologic Society, vice president of the Texas Dermatologic Society, and chairman of the board of directors of the American College of Cryosurgery.

In 1996 Dr. Limmer received the Platinum Follicle Award, presented annually to one individual by the International Society of Hair Restoration

Surgery for the most important basic research in hair anatomy and physiology in the world.

Robert E. McClellan, M.D.
9911 West Pico Blvd.
Los Angeles, CA 90035
(310) 553-9113

- Surgeon/Board Certified by the American Board of Surgery

Dr. McClellan received his medical degree from the University of Utah School of Medicine in 1975. His internship in surgery was at Providence Hospital in Southfield, Michigan.

From 1976 to 1978 he served as a medical doctor and regimental surgeon for the U.S. Navy, stationed in Okinawa, Japan, and in Brunswick, Maine.

Dr. McClellan did his residency in general surgery at Berkshire Medical Center in Pittsfield, Massachusetts. He served as instructor in general surgery at the University of Massachusetts Medical School.

Dr. McClellan practiced general surgery from 1982 to 1988 in Utah and Wyoming. He has been practicing hair transplantation full time since then.

O'Tar Norwood, M.D.
5710 N. Portland, #310
Oklahoma City, OK 73112
(405) 951-4970

- Dermatologist/Board Certified by the American Board of Dermatology
- Associate Clinical Professor of Dermatology, University of Oklahoma Health Sciences Center

Dr. Norwood's name is perhaps the most well known among balding men, since he set the standard for classifying degrees of male pattern baldness with the Norwood Scale. His study "Male Pattern Baldness Classification Incidence," first published in a medical journal in 1975, became a classic and remains the standard today. It is used by all hair-transplant surgeons and physicians from all over the world.

Dr. Norwood has more than thirty published articles to his credit and is sought after as a teacher and lecturer. He is cofounder of the International Society for Hair Restoration Surgery and was the founder, editor, and publisher of the bimonthly publication *Hair Transplant Forum International.*

He graduated from the University of Arkansas in 1953, then received his doctor of medicine degree from the University of Arkansas Medical School in 1957.

Dr. Norwood served in the U.S. Navy for three years, interning at the U.S. Navy Hospital in Oakland, California.

He did his residency in dermatology at the University of Oklahoma from 1961 to 1964.

Dr. Norwood has been extremely active in numerous professional societies and has held many offices, including president of the Oklahoma State Dermatological Association.

He publishes regularly in medical journals, including the *Journal of Dermatologic Surgery* and *Dermatologic Surgery and Oncology.*

Bernard P. Nusbaum, M.D.
7867 S.W. 88th St.
Miami, FL 33156
(305) 274-2202

- Dermatologist/Board Certified by the American Board of Dermatology

Dr. Nusbaum has been widely published in the fields of dermatology and hair transplantation and has been extremely active in research and professional societies. He is in demand as a lecturer and has presented dozens of programs, research findings, and clinical reports at medical conferences.

He graduated from the University of Colorado in 1974, then received his doctor of medicine degree from the University of Miami School of Medicine in 1979.

Dr. Nusbaum interned in internal medicine at Mount Sinai Medical Center in Miami Beach from 1979 to 1980. He did his residency in dermatology at Mount Sinai from 1980 to 1983, serving as chief resident in dermatology from 1981 to 1983. He has been a clinical assistant professor lecturing in dermatology in the Department of Family Medicine at the University of Miami School of Medicine and has also been a clinical instructor at the Department of Dermatology and Cutaneous Surgery at the University of Miami School of Medicine.

His published articles in medical journals include "Hair Transplantation: A Three-Stage Approach for Creating the Hairline" in the *Journal of Dermatologic Surgery and Oncology* (1992), among a dozen others. In *Hair Transplant Forum International* he has published "Hair Transplantation in Black Patients" (1991) and "Frontal Forelock: Overall Design" (1995).

William R. Rassman, M.D.
9911 West Pico Blvd.
Los Angeles, CA 90035
(310) 553-6790

- Surgeon/Board Certified by the American Board of Surgery

With Robert M. Bernstein, M.D., Dr. Rassman pioneered the follicular-transplantation method of hair transplantation (see Chapter Four).

Dr. Rassman received his medical degree from

the Medical College of Virginia in 1966. He completed his surgical internship at the University of Minnesota and later became a cardiac fellow under Dr. C. W. Lillehei. He completed his residency in general surgery at Cornell and Dartmouth Medical Centers. From 1969 to 1971 Dr. Rassman served in the U.S. Army as a surgeon. He was stationed in Kentucky and in the Republic of Vietnam. During his tour of duty he was awarded the Silver Star and earned the rank of major.

Dr. Rassman did major research in the cardiac field and commercialized the Intra-Aortic Balloon Pump in 1969, a device credited today with saving thousands of lives each year. Dr. Rassman continues to be active in the cardiac field.

He has patents in numerous fields, from computer software to biotechnology. In the hair-transplant field he has pioneered new techniques and invented the Hair Densitometer™, which measures hair density and the health of the hair.

Dr. Rassman is a frequently published author in peer-reviewed medical journals, and he presents scientific papers before national and international societies.

Paul T. Rose, M.D.
6140 Bayside Drive
New Port Richey, FL 34652
(813) 848-7229

- Dermatologist/Board Certified by the American Board of Dermatology
- Assistant Clinical Professor at the University of South Florida in the Department of Medicine, Division of Dermatology

Dr. Rose received his medical degree from the State University of New York at Downstate Medical Center in Brooklyn, New York, in 1979. He completed an internal medicine internship in 1980 at the University of Connecticut Medical Center in Farmington, Connecticut. In 1988 Dr. Rose completed his residency in dermatology at Temple University Skin and Cancer Hospital in Philadelphia, Pennsylvania.

He has given several presentations on hair restoration to prestigious societies, including a "Live Surgery Workshop for Hair Transplantation" for the American Academy of Cosmetic Surgery.

Dr. Rose has published several articles in the field of micrographic surgery and continues to do research and write in this field.

Ron Shapiro, M.D.
3023 Eastland Blvd., #113
Clearwater, FL 33761
(888) 741-1110

- Internist/Board Certified in Internal Medicine

- Also Board Certified by the American Board of Emergency Medicine

Dr. Shapiro graduated from Emory University in 1975 and received his doctor of medicine degree from Emory University School of Medicine in 1979.

He interned in internal medicine at Emanuel Hospital in Portland, Oregon, from 1979 to 1980. He did his residency in internal medicine there from 1980 to 1982. He also trained in surgical and trauma emergency medicine at Harbor General Hospital in Torrance, California, in 1981 and in pediatric emergency medicine at Grady Memorial Hospital in Atlanta, Georgia, in 1982.

Dr. Shapiro is active in professional societies and research, and he has presented lectures on hair transplantation at medical conferences in the United States and abroad, including live surgery lectures in the U.S. and Rome.

He has published research papers and articles in medical journals and publications.

Bradley R. Wolf, M.D.
11821 Mason Montgomery Road
Cincinnati, OH 45249
(513) 774–0400

- Surgeon/Board Certified in Emergency Medicine

Dr. Wolf practices exclusively as a hair transplant surgeon. He received his Doctor of Medicine degree from Indiana University School of Medicine in 1980, and did his internship in General Surgery at Eastern Virginia Graduate School of Medicine in Norfolk, Virginia, from 1980–1981. He then did his residency in General Surgery there from 1981–1982.

Dr. Wolf is a member of a number of professional associations, and has lectured extensively on hair transplantation surgery at medical conferences in the U.S., Europe and Russia.

He has also presented live surgery workshops at medical conferences in the U.S. and Russia.

Subscribe to The Bald Truth Journal™

Now that science has identified the cause of male pattern baldness, advances in hair-loss prevention and restoration are being made more rapidly than ever.

The Bald Truth Journal, a quarterly newsletter published by Spencer David Kobren, is the only unbiased, objective patient/consumer guide available, since it has no product or physician sponsorship.

Each issue includes the latest research on drug therapies and natural treatments; state-of-the-art techniques and advances in hair-transplantation surgery; physician updates and interviews; reviews of other hair products and hair systems; and the experiences of our readers.

It is important to be armed with this information. Too many people have made bad choices simply because they were uninformed or misinformed.

You can continue to keep up to date with your $29.95 subscription. To subscribe by mail:

The Bald Truth Journal
500 East 77th St., Suite 1608
New York, NY 10021

Or phone:

(800) 446-5954

Pavillion Harvest

The author now makes available a standardized combination of the most effective DHT-inhibiting herbs—saw palmetto, *Pygeum africanum,* and stinging nettle—in one capsule, formulated at the clinically recommended potency levels.

Pavillion Harvest also offers Green Tea extract.

Call Pavillion Harvest to order: (800) 446-5954.

ABOUT THE AUTHOR

Spencer David Kobren is the country's most prominent and effective hair loss consumer/patient advocate, and the Founder and Director of The Bald Truth Foundation, the only organization dedicated to consumer advocacy, education and funding research regarding hair loss.

He is also host of "The Bald Truth," his nationally syndicated weekly radio program; a feature columnist on three of the most respected hair-loss Web sites, including *regrowth.com;* and has his own Web site: *www.thebald truth.org.*

After years of researching hair loss and finally overcoming the early stages of his own male pattern baldness, which began a dozen years ago at age 22, he has dedicated himself to helping others prevent and treat hair loss. As a consumer advocate, he consults on issues of patient and consumer rights in this unregulated industry.

Kobren and his work are the focus of the Discovery Channel documentary also titled "The Bald Truth" and have been featured in articles in many publications, including *GQ, The Wall Street Journal, Men's Health,* and *The New York Times.*

He lives in New York City.

Printed in the United States
By Bookmasters